M000015077

Measurements for Long-Term Care

To the authors of instruments,
whose work makes it possible
to improve the quality of long-term care

Measurements for Long-Term Care

A GUIDEBOOK FOR NURSES

Sarah R. Beaton & Susan A. Voge

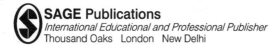

SAGE Publications
International Educational and Professional Publisher
Thousand Oaks   London   New Delhi

For information:

SAGE Publications, Inc.
2455 Teller Road
Thousand Oaks, California 91320
E-mail: order@sagepub.com

SAGE Publications Ltd.
6 Bonhill Street
London EC2A 4PU
United Kingdom

SAGE Publications India Pvt. Ltd.
M-32 Market
Greater Kailash I
New Delhi 110 048 India

Printed in the United States of America
Library of Congress Cataloging-in-Publication Data

Beaton, Sarah R.
    Measurements for long-term care / Sarah R.
      Beaton and Susan A. Voge.
      p.   cm.
    Includes bibliographical references and index.
    ISBN 0-8039-5388-7 (cloth: acid-free paper)
      1. Long-term care of the sick—Research—Methodology. 2. Nursing
home care—Research—Methodology.   I. Voge, Susan A.   II. Title.
RT120.L64B4   1998
362.1'6'072—dc21   97-33870

98 99 00 01 02 03 10 7 6 5 4 3 2 1

Acquiring Editor:	Dan Ruth
Editorial Assistant:	Anna Howland
Production Editor:	Diana E. Axelsen
Production Assistant:	Lynn Miyata
Typesetter/Designer:	Christina M. Hill
Cover Designer:	Ravi Balasuriya
Print Buyer:	Anna Chin

Contents

Preface

This book has its origins in a collaboration between a nurse and a librarian, an interdisciplinary partnership of faculty members that we heartily endorse. We are grateful for assistance from many quarters. First, we thank the authors of the instruments reviewed. They have been very generous about sharing their work. We are grateful to nursing and library colleagues who provided reviews and suggestions. Sage reviewers and the editorial board made helpful comments. Members of the editorial board were Elaine J. Amella, Jean Bresnahan, Cheryl Dellasega, Mary Duffy, Jacqueline Picciano, and Sharon Weinberg. A Professional Staff Congress/City University of New York award to Susan Voge helped to defray costs. We especially appreciate the patience and skill of editors Christine Smedley, Dan Ruth, and Diana Axelsen.

Introduction

Nurses engaged in practice and research in long-term care need to describe groups of patients, measure outcomes, and operationalize research and clinical variables. To accomplish these and other measurement goals, they need access to instruments (also called *measures, scales, tools,* or *tests*). This guidebook is intended as a reference for instrument acquisition. The aim has been to provide readers with preliminary information sufficient to allow them to choose an instrument for subsequent study.

We believe that nursing practice in long-term care can be improved with the use of measuring instruments. Thus, this book was written for nurses and nursing students who want to (a) raise the level of inquiry in nursing practice, (b) document the effectiveness of interventions, (c) improve communication in interdisciplinary environments, (d) compare clinical outcomes and research results between settings and over time, (e) increase confidence in decision making, (f) unite practice with research, and (g) participate in the further development of the North American Nursing Diagnosis Association (NANDA) taxonomy.

In addition to their use in research and practice, instruments can facilitate learning. They can be used as outlines for assessments. A student learning to assess for delirium, for example, could use the Neecham Confusion Scale or the Confusion Assessment Method to recognize delirium. What better way to understand the symptoms associated with anxiety than to study the Anxiety Status Inventory or the Taylor Manifest Anxiety Scale? Training to use instruments can also sharpen observation skills and interviewing techniques.

Conceptual Frameworks

Nurses practicing in long-term care make a unique contribution and are also members of an interdisciplinary team. The roles for professional nurses in long-term care may be guided by two broad frameworks. The first was described by Morse (1992), who stated that "the ultimate purpose of nursing is to promote comfort" (p. 92). She wrote of patient-centered nursing and called for studies that describe nursing practice at the micro level as well as investigations of the efficacy of nursing practice in terms of reduced morbidity and mortality. The instruments described in this book can assist nurses who are interested in both these levels. The second framework is drawn from the American Nurses' Association (ANA) Social Policy Statement (ANA, 1980), in which the definition of nursing was related to ANA standards of nursing practice, including nursing research, and to the steps of the nursing process, including nursing diagnosis and outcome measurement.

Definitions

The term *long-term care* has traditionally referred to care in nursing homes. For this book, the definition of long-term care includes preventive, supportive, maintenance, diagnostic, therapeutic, and rehabilitative services delivered in institutions, home health agencies, support programs, foster homes, day hospitals, day care programs, senior citizens' centers, and rehabilitation programs. Although children and young adults also receive long-term care services, the older adult population is the primary focus of this book.

The nursing services to which this book can refer were described by Lang, Kraegel, Rantz, and Krejci (1990). They include health promotion, health teaching, disease prevention, health screening, health care management, the fostering of self-care, client and family support, actual physical and mental care, and administration of medical treatments.

In this book, the term *patient* describes persons whom others have come to call *clients, residents,* and *participants.*

Selection Criteria

How were instruments in this book selected? They were relevant to long-term care nursing and had an adequate developmental history with an initial published report, plus information about at least one subsequent study. They looked promising for describing patients and/or measuring outcomes. Each of the instruments was feasible for administration by nurses and was accessible.

Entries reflect the interdisciplinary environment of long-term care. We searched for relevant materials in the nursing research literature and the multidisciplinary long-term care research literature, to which nurses contribute. We used the same databases and other sources recommended to the reader in the next section of this book, "How to Update Test Information or Find New Instruments."

The relevance of entries to nursing practice was verified by comparing them with a list of the "top 20" nursing diagnoses prevalent in long-term care facilities (Fielding et al., 1997) and with estimates of prevalence in home care (Keating, 1988). To verify accessibility, we ourselves obtained each tool either through library acquisition or through contact with authors.

The variety of domains for entries defied any single categorical system. Therefore, we have assembled them alphabetically and provided indexes for abbreviations and acronyms, authors, titles, subject terms, and nursing diagnoses. The nursing diagnoses index is based on NANDA's 1996 publication, *NANDA Nursing Diagnoses: Definitions and Classification (1997-1998)*. There is a glossary to assist readers with terminology used in the entries that may be obscure.

About the Entries

Each of the more than 100 entries in this book includes the title, name(s) of author(s), address of primary author (in most cases), a short description of the instrument, brief summaries of psychometric properties, procedures, sample item(s), information about scoring, the sources for the tool, and references. The information provided is based on the literature and on written and oral communications with instrument authors. We have not attempted to compare instruments.

We considered the advantages and disadvantages of including copies of tools in this book and decided against this approach. Using instruments to measure variables in long-term care is a complex intellectual task, a process not to be taken lightly. This book is intended only as a first-step reference book, a sourcebook to help the reader get started. To confirm instrument selection, a user needs documentation far beyond the brief information reported in this book. A copy of an instrument is only part of the information needed. More detail about instrument development and the theoretical framework for the instrument will be available in publications by the authors. Authors will need to be contacted for administration and scoring instructions; up-to-the-minute information about the instrument's reliability, validity, and sensitivity; and possible revisions or modified versions.

When users want to reproduce or quote from an instrument, they need permission from copyright holders. Some authors hold copyrights for their instruments. In most cases, however, copyrights are held by the publishers of the journal in which the instrument was initially reported.

Perhaps the most important reason for contact with authors is their continuing interest in the use of their instruments.

Authors' addresses can get out of date quickly. Mail or phone calls to academic settings can be fruitful. If other sources are needed, professional directories can be used. The *Directory of Nurse Researchers* (published by Sigma Theta Tau) and the *National Faculty Directory* (published by Gale Research) are two examples. Some online databases, such as those described in the next section of this book, also list the address of the first author. With Internet access, one may now search for individuals. Two resources are "WhoWhere" and the Internet "White Pages." They allow searching for personal names to find addresses, phone numbers, and e-mail addresses.

Choosing an Instrument

Choosing a measure depends on the purposes of the clinician/investigator. An instrument is never ideal for every purpose or setting. Each is a work in progress, evolving as results are reported about its use by other clinicians and researchers. Tools suitable for measurement in clinical practice may not work well for intervention research (Kane, 1993). Users have the responsibility of evaluating the instruments they select. Strickland (1994) outlined 32 questions one can answer to evaluate an existing instrument. Among many criteria that clinicians and researchers use when choosing an instrument are the classic issues of validity, reliability, sensitivity, and feasibility for administration and scoring. Readers are cautioned to note that many instruments have not been shown to have sensitivity: That is, the extent to which they can detect change is unknown. Therefore, they may not be useful in demonstrating the efficacy of nursing interventions (Stewart & Archbold, 1992, 1993).

Users of instruments need to be familiar with the constructs inherent in measurement. For more detailed information than can be provided in a glossary, texts such as Polit and Hungler's *Nursing Research: Principles and*

Methods and the "Focus on Psychometrics" features appearing in the journal *Research in Nursing and Health* are excellent resources.

For long-term care, additional measurement issues must be considered (Matteson, 1985). Among these are brevity, reading levels, sensory alterations, medications, pain, living in an institution, slowed reaction times, and the extreme care that elders may take in responding. Brevity should be considered not only because of the potential for fatigue but also for possible iatrogenic effects of testing itself. Pfeffer, Kurosaki, Harrah, Chance, and Filos (1982) pointed out the need to be brief enough "to minimize distress that might be aroused in a spouse, friend, or relative by an extended recital of incapacity" (p. 324). One can assume that such recitals would have effects on patients as well. It is important to consider the ethical issues involved in the use of any measurement technique (Cassel, 1988).

Just as a single instrument is a work in progress, so too, a compendium of instruments is subject to revision and change. This book is an effort to put preliminary information about instruments for long-term care in the hands of nurses. Nurses themselves will need to add the deliberative process that will make the effort fully relevant to their own practice and research.

How to Proceed With Instruments

To select an instrument, the reader should perform the following steps:

1. Consult this book's indexes as needed.
2. Read an entry in this book or in another compendium or database.
3. Search the literature to update for other references, using information in "How to Update Test Information or Find New Instruments" in the next section of this book.
4. Analyze original sources tracing the instrument's evolution.
5. Confirm that work on the instrument is anchored in a theory congruent with your model for practice or research.
6. Contact the author to obtain a copy of the latest version of the instrument and gain permission for use. If the literature is abundant and if a copy is available in the public domain, this step may not be necessary.
7. Prepare to administer the instrument by reviewing it carefully. Many instruments require specific training and practice before administration. *Every* instrument requires careful review so that the reliability of observations will be facilitated.
8. Pilot-test before administration.

References

American Nurses' Association. (1980). *Nursing: A social policy statement.* Washington, DC: Author.

Cassel, C. K. (1988). Ethical issues in the conduct of research in long-term care. *Gerontologist, 28*(Suppl.), 90-96.

Fielding, J., Beaton, S., Baier, L., Rallis, D., Ryan, R. M., & Siripornsawan, D. (1997). Nursing diagnoses and related outcome objectives for long-term care. In M. J. Rantz & P. LeMone (Eds.), *Classification of nursing diagnoses: Proceedings of the 12th conference.* Glendale, CA: CINAHL Information Systems.

Kane, R. L. (1993). The implications of assessment. *Journal of Gerontology, 48,* 27-31.

Keating, S. B. (1988). The measurement of client outcomes in home health care agencies. In C. F. Waltz & O. L. Strickland (Eds.), *Measurement of nursing outcomes: Vol. 1. Measuring client outcomes* (pp. 457-471). New York: Springer.

Lang, N. M., Kraegel, J. M., Rantz, M. J., & Krejci, J. W. (1990). *Quality of health care for older people: A review of nursing studies.* Kansas City, MO: American Nurses Association.

Matteson, M. A. (1985). Measuring gerontological nursing's impact on the elderly. *Journal of Gerontological Nursing, 11*(6), 28-33.

Morse, J. M. (1992). Comfort. *Clinical Nursing Research, 1,* 91-108.

North American Nursing Diagnoses Association. (1996). *NANDA nursing diagnosis: Definitions and classification (1997-1998).* Philadelphia: Author.

Pfeffer, R. I., Kurosaki, T. T., Harrah, C. H., Chance, J. M., & Filos, S. (1982). Measurement of functional activities in older adults in the community. *Journal of Gerontology, 37,* 323-329.

Stewart, B. J., & Archbold, P. G. (1992). Nursing intervention studies require outcome measures that are sensitive to change: Part one. *Research in Nursing and Health, 15,* 477-481.

Stewart, B. J., & Archbold, P. G. (1993). Nursing intervention studies require outcome measures that are sensitive to change: Part two. *Research in Nursing and Health, 16,* 77-81.

Strickland, O. (1994). Using existing instruments. *Journal of Nursing Measurement, 2,* 3-6.

How to Update Test Information
or Find New Instruments

The most important resource for someone interested in information about instruments is a reference librarian. Information sources change rapidly. There are many resources available in libraries.

The Cumulative Index to Nursing and Allied Health, or CINAHL, is the only database designed specifically to meet the information needs of nurses and allied health professionals. It is the database equivalent of the print version of the *Cumulative Index to Nursing and Allied Health Literature.* CINAHL provides access to virtually all English-language nursing journals, publications from the American Nurses' Association and the National League for Nursing, and primary journals from 13 allied health disciplines. About half of the records include abstracts. Since 1991, CINAHL has been indexing nursing dissertations; in 1992, they began indexing proceedings, book chapters, and pamphlets. In 1996, they began including all the references listed in articles and records about instruments. Twenty-five instrument records were added in the first 6 months. Some of these records include the full texts of tools. CINAHL expects to continue adding new instrument records.

MEDLINE, produced by the U.S. National Library of Medicine, represents worldwide coverage of the biomedical literature from 1966 to the present, indexing more than 3,700 journals. MEDLINE includes all articles indexed for the *International Nursing Index,* which is published separately in print form. The *International Nursing Index* covers nursing journals as well as articles subject-headed for nursing in other National Library of Medicine indexes. Text of the articles is not provided, but approximately half of the records have abstracts written by the articles' authors.

The Health and Psychosocial Instruments, or HAPI CD (published by Behavioral Measurement Database Services), covers research instruments about health, nursing, psychology, behavioral science, business, and library science. Most have been published since 1985. Less well-known and otherwise difficult-to-find instruments are emphasized. The database contains more than 25,000 records. HAPI indexes the study in which the instrument was used initially, subsequent studies for which the instrument was used when possible, selected psychometric data, and the source of the instrument. New instruments are added from regular scans of approximately 300 journals and selectively from test publishers' catalogues, *Dissertation Abstracts,* and conference proceedings. HAPI is available only as a CD; contact Evelyn Perloff, Director, Behavioral Measurement Database Services, P.O. Box 110287, Pittsburgh, PA 15232-0787, telephone (412) 687-6850.

The Mental Measurements Yearbook (MMY) CD (published by Silver-Platter Information) contains descriptive information and critical reviews for more than 1,800 commercially available standardized educational, personality, vocational aptitude, psychological, and related English-language tests. It covers the years from 1989 to the present and is updated twice a year. Information on each test includes name, classification, author(s), publisher, publication date, price, time requirements, existence of validity and reliability data, score descriptions, levels and intended populations, and critical reviews. It is available both as a CD and online.

The *Mental Measurements Yearbook (MMY)* print series has been published since 1938, with the older volumes available in most large libraries. Another publication, *Tests in Print,* indexes all the editions of *MMY* and also serves as a comprehensive bibliography for all known commercially available English-language tests currently in print. The most recent edition at this writing is *Tests in Print IV* (Murphy, Conoley, & Impara, 1994).

Tests: A Comprehensive Reference for Assessments in Psychology, Education, and Business provides in its most recent (third) edition (Sweetland & Keyser, 1991) concise descriptions of more than 3,000 published tests, including populations targeted, purposes, methods of administration, and publication information.

Dissertation Abstracts Online provides summaries of doctoral theses from around the world published since 1981 and master's theses published since 1988. Tests are often mentioned in the abstracts and can be searched by name.

Psychological Abstracts (PA) scans more than 1,400 journals in the social and behavioral sciences. Selected sources from related disciplines, such as biology, education, management, medicine, psychiatry, social work, and sociology, are also included in *PA*. Electronic access to *Psychological Abstracts,* called PsycInfo, covers the literature back through 1887. PsycInfo also indexes English-language books and book chapters published worldwide since 1987. Except for the oldest materials, all entries include abstracts.

The AgeLine database is produced by the American Association of Retired Persons (AARP) and provides bibliographic coverage of social gerontology, the study of aging in social, psychological, health-related, and economic contexts. The delivery of health care for the older population and its associated costs and policies are particularly well covered.

OCLC Online Computer Library Center, Inc., maintains a union catalogue of the holdings of more than 9,000 libraries worldwide. In many academic libraries, this database, called WorldCat, is available for searching on a user-friendly system called First Search. Most books, videotapes, computer programs, and other publications about any subject, including testing and measurement, can be identified using this system. When the material is not available in a "home" academic or public library, patrons can gain access to material found in WorldCat through interlibrary loan systems.

HealthSTAR is a bibliographic database from the National Library of Medicine and the American Hospital Association, containing citations—and abstracts for half the records—of the literature dealing with the clinical and nonclinical aspects of health care delivery. The database cites journal articles, monographs, technical reports, meeting abstracts and papers, book chapters, government documents, and newspaper articles from 1975 to the present. Among the topics emphasized in this database are the evaluation of patient outcomes and the effectiveness of procedures, programs, products, services, and processes.

The Sociofile database contains information from approximately 2,000 journals in 30 different languages from about 55 countries. It covers sociology and related disciplines by including bibliographic citations and abstracts and enhanced dissertation citations.

Social SciSearch (SSCI) is a multidisciplinary database indexing every significant item from the 1,500 social science journals considered most important throughout the world and from social science articles selected from 3,000 additional journals in the natural, physical, and biomedical sciences. It belongs to a family of indexes and databases that permits searching of articles by cited reference. These indexes are a source that allows the user to search in the direction from past writing to present literature. Obtaining current citations to past writings about an instrument is one way to update. The SSCI database is a good source for information about instruments that have continued to be reported in the literature. A drawback to the citation databases is some limitation in the number of journals scanned for references. For example, only 14 nursing journals are scanned in the SSCI. The citation databases are unlimited in the sources cited, however, which include books and reports in addition to articles.

Commercial Publishers

Commercial or published tests may be sold through test-publishing companies. They may have been first published in a journal article but later made available commercially. The publications *MMY* and *Tests* (Sweetland & Keyser, 1991) give current addresses and phone numbers for test publishers. Many have toll-free phone numbers. It is important to call before ordering because some publishers restrict purchases. For example, tests such as the Beck Depression Index or the Beck Hopelessness Scale may be available only to psychologists, individuals with PhDs, or those who have had course work in psychometrics. When students want access to these tests, they may need to order them through a faculty member or other qualified contact person.

Unpublished tests are usually discovered through literature searches in which tests are named in articles or dissertation abstracts. Another printed source for unpublished tests is the *Directory of Unpublished Experimental Mental Measures* (published by Human Sciences Press from 1974 to 1985 and by William C. Brown after 1985).

How to Search Databases

Enter words or phrases to describe your topic. Two or more concepts may be crossed using the *and* connector. Topics may also be searched by using the list of subject terms established for the particular database, usually found in the thesaurus for that database, either published or online.

Fortunately, most database entries include abstracts, which often include names of research instruments when they have been used. Instruments are not usually mentioned in titles, however, and few databases list them as subject or index terms. CINAHL is the pioneer in this area. Since 1991, this database has included a subject field for listing instruments mentioned in an article. A keyword or unlimited word search will work best in searches for articles reporting use of instruments.

Where to Find Databases

Online retrieval of information is available in various ways. You can visit a library, usually a large public library or an academic or health institution library, to use electronic sources of information. Some databases (PsycInfo, MEDLINE) are available at most large libraries. More specialized databases are found only at libraries serving patrons with specific needs for them (CINAHL, Dissertation Abstracts, HAPI, MMY). The high cost of the Social Sciences Citation Index (SSCI) has meant that it is available only at the largest university and public research libraries. The *Gale Directory of Databases* (published by Gale Research biannually) keeps track of how databases are accessed. This publication itself is also available electronically and is updated twice a year.

Increasingly, information databases are becoming available on the Internet, giving individuals many more options for searching them. At the time of this writing, one provider, HealthGate, has made MEDLINE available and free to anyone in the world. The ERIC (Educational Resources Information Center of the U.S. Department of Education) Clearinghouse on Assessment and Evaluation, based at the Education Department of the Catholic University of America, maintains a Web site allowing open access to some test resources at http://ericae.net. For example, the Buros Test Review Locator provides references to reviews and descriptions of tests in either the *MMY* or *Tests in Print.* Another resource at this Web site is the Educational Testing Service (ETS) Test File. This Test Collection database contains records on more than 10,000 tests and research instruments that describe the instruments and provide availability information. It also references the ETS's *Tests on Microfiche,* which provides full-text reproduction of measures with manuals and scoring information. A test publisher, Pro-Ed, maintains two databases at this site. The Pro-Ed Test Review Database tells you which volumes of *Test Critiques* (Keyser & Sweetland, 1984-1994) contain reviews of the test you have identified. The critiques offer the reader practical applications and uses, settings in which the test is used, appropriate as well as inappropriate subjects, and guidelines for administration, scoring, and interpretation. They cite normative data, validity and reliability information, and expert opinions about a test. A final feature of each review is the critique portion, which summarizes and reviews the instrument. Also available here is the Pro-Ed Test Publisher Locator, which contains the last known address of 470 major test publishers.

Watch the Internet for new resources about measurement in long-term care. Joyce A. Post, the librarian at the Philadelphia Geriatric Center, publishes an ongoing column about Internet and e-mail resources on aging. Her files may be accessed at two addresses: http://www.aoa.dhhs.gov/aoa/pages/ jpostlst.html and http://www.geron.org.

Other Sources of Information About Instruments

Division of Clinical Research, National Institute of Mental Health. (1988). Assessment in diagnosis and treatment of geropsychiatric patients. *Psychopharmacology Bulletin, 24*(4). A special issue of this journal providing comprehensive coverage of instrumentation in the field of geropsychiatry.

Fischer, J., & Corcoran, K. (1994). *Measures for clinical practice: A sourcebook* (2nd ed., Vols. 1-2). New York: Free Press. Reprints over 300 self-report measures containing fewer than 50 questions.

Frank-Stromborg, M., & Olsen, S. J. (Eds.). (1997). *Instruments for health-care research.* Boston: Jones and Bartlett. Review instruments for use by nurses and other health care researchers.

Gallo, J. J., Reichel, W., & Andersen, L. (1988). *Handbook of geriatric assessment.* Gaithersburg, MD: Aspen. This book emphasizes material that has practical application in primary care settings.

Groth-Marnat, G. (1990). *Handbook of psychological assessment* (2nd ed.). New York: John Wiley. A handbook about tests.

Hersen, M., & Bellack, A. S. (Eds.). (1988). *Dictionary of behavioral assessment techniques.* Elmsford, NY: Pergamon. A handbook for psychological testing methods, such as the visual analogue scale.

Kane, R. A., & Kane, R. L. (1981). *Assessing the elderly.* Lexington, MA: D. C. Heath. This volume covers approximately 86 instruments; many pertain to long-term care.

Lawton, M. P., & Teresi, J. A. (Eds.). (1994). Focus on assessment techniques. *Annual Review of Gerontology and Geriatrics, 14.* This volume provides 16 chapters about assessment techniques written by experts; most are related to long-term care.

Mangen, D. J., & Peterson, W. A. (1982-1984). *Research instruments in social gerontology* (Vols. 1-3). Minneapolis: University of Minnesota Press. Includes reviews of 400 measures, many fully reprinted, on clinical and social psychology (Vol. 1), social roles and participation (Vol. 2), and health, program evaluation, and demography (Vol. 3). Lists instruments not included in this book.

Matteson, M. A., McConnell, E. S., & Linton, A. D. (1997). *Gerontological nursing: Concepts and practice* (2nd ed.). Philadelphia: W. B. Saunders. This textbook includes copies of many instruments relevant to long-term care.

McDowell, I., & Newell, C. (1996). *Measuring health: A guide to rating scales and questionnaires* (2nd ed.). New York: Oxford University Press. Provides copies of over 80 sociomedical measurement methods covering topics including physical disability and handicap, social health, psychological well-being, depression, mental status testing, pain measurement, general health status, and quality of life.

Miller, D. C. (1991). *Handbook of research design and social measurement* (5th ed.). Newbury Park, CA: Sage. Summarizes sociologically oriented research instruments and reprints about 25 full measures, such as Neal and Seeman's Powerlessness Scale.

Robinson, J. P., Shaver, P. R., & Wright, J. M. (1991). *Measures of personality and social psychological attitude* (2nd ed.). San Diego: Academic Press. Reviews 150 attitude measures in social psychology and includes copies of many, such as Version 3 of the UCLA Loneliness Scale.

Schutte, N. S., & Malouff, J. M. (1995). *Sourcebook of adult assessment strategies.* New York: Plenum. Includes copies of approximately 70 instruments.

Ward, M. J., & Lindeman, C. A. (1979). *Instruments for measuring nursing practice and other health care variables* (Vols. 1-2). Hyattsville, MD: U.S. Health Resources Administration, Division of Nursing. (Also available as ERIC Document Reproduction Service No. ED 171 763.) This early nursing collection reproduced 135 psychosocial instruments, such as the Health Locus of Control Scale.

References

Keyser, D. J., & Sweetland, R. C. (Eds.). (1984-1994). *Test critiques* (Vols. 1-10). Austin, TX: Pro-Ed.

Murphy, L. L., Conoley, J. C., & Impara, J. C. (Eds.). (1994). *Tests in print IV (TIP IV): An index to tests, test reviews, and the literature on specific tests* (Vols. 1-2). Lincoln: University of Nebraska-Lincoln, Buros Institute of Mental Measurements.

Sweetland, R. C., & Keyser, D. J. (1991). *Tests: A comprehensive reference for assessments in psychology, education, and business* (3rd ed.). Austin, TX: Pro-Ed.

Additional Suggested Readings

Anastasi, A. (1988). *Psychological testing* (6th ed.). New York: Macmillan.

ERIC Clearinghouse on Tests, Measurement, and Evaluation. (1989). *Glossary of measurement terms, Digest EDO-TM-89-1.* Washington, DC: Author.

Reed, J. G., & Baxter, P. M. (1992). *Library use: A handbook for psychology* (2nd ed.). Washington, DC: American Psychological Association.

ABNORMAL INVOLUNTARY MOVEMENT SCALE (AIMS)

AUTHOR: National Institute of Mental Health (NIMH)
ADDRESS: Psychopharmacology Research Branch
            National Institute of Mental Health
            Division of Clinical Treatment Research
            5600 Fishers Lane, Room 18-105
            Rockville, MD 20857

DESCRIPTION: The Abnormal Involuntary Movement Scale (AIMS) is a 12-item tool designed to screen for tardive dyskinesia (TD) by systematically assessing for movements of the face, lips, perioral area, jaw, tongue, upper and lower extremities, and trunk. The examiner makes judgments about the severity of movements and the degree to which they are incapacitating. Users of the AIMS are cautioned not to consider severity ratings as equivalent to a diagnosis of TD and are advised to consult Schooler and Kane (1982) and Woerner et al. (1991). Specific detailed examination procedures are an integral part of the AIMS. One cannot administer the AIMS without following these procedures. The NIMH staff have also developed instructions for videotaping the AIMS exam.

PSYCHOMETRIC PROPERTIES: Whall, Engle, Edwards, Bobel, and Haberland (1983) developed a screening program for TD. Four RNs who were trained for the project, a neurological clinical specialist, and a neurologist participated. Paired RN raters assessed 60 nursing home residents independently. Correlations of agreement between raters for AIMS items were significant at $p < 0.05$ and ranged from 0.59 for "the lips and perioral area" to 0.97 for "patient's awareness of abnormal movements." These investigators also showed that the AIMS examination procedures were acceptable to subjects.

PROCEDURE: The patient is observed unobtrusively at rest either before or after the examination. A hard, firm chair without arms is used in the examination. Before testing begins, the examiner asks the patient whether there is anything in his or her mouth and, if so, to remove it. There is an inquiry about condition of teeth and whether the subject wears dentures. The examiner then proceeds to follow 10 further steps in a systematic way. The examination is completed before any recordings are made on the AIMS form.

SAMPLE ITEM: "Ask patient whether he/she notices any movements in mouth, face, hands or feet. If yes, ask to describe and to what extent they currently bother or interfere with his/her activities" (NIMH, 1974, p. 2).

SCORING: Each item is rated on a 5-point scale. Instructions read, "Rate the highest severity observed. Rate movements that occur upon activation one *less* than those observed spontaneously" (NIMH, 1974, p. 1).

SOURCE: The instrument and the examination procedure are reprinted in Avorn (1989). These materials plus guidelines for a procedure to videotape the AIMS are available from NIMH, telephone (301) 443-4513. Directions for administration are outlined in Guy (1976). The AIMS is in the public domain.

REFERENCES

Avorn, J. (1989). Abnormal Involuntary Movement Scale (AIMS). *Psychopharmacological Bulletin, 24,* 781-783.

Guy, W. (Ed.). (1976). *Early Clinical Drug Evaluation Unit assessment manual for psychopharmacology* (Rev. ed., DHEW Pub. No. ADM 76-338). Washington, DC: U.S. Department of Health, Education and Welfare.

National Institute of Mental Health. (1974). *Abnormal Involuntary Movement Scale* (Form MH 9-117). (Available from the author at address listed above)

Schooler, N. R., & Kane, J. M. (1982). Research diagnosis for tardive dyskinesia. *Archives of General Psychiatry, 30,* 486-487.

Whall, A. L., Engle, V., Edwards, A., Bobel, L., & Haberland, C. (1983). Development of a screening program for tardive dyskinesia: Feasibility issues. *Nursing Research, 32,* 151-156.

Woerner, W. G., Kane, J. M., Lieberman, J. A., Alvir, J., Bergmann, K. J., Borenstein, M., Schooler, N. R., Mukherjee, S., Rotrosen, J., Rubenstein, M., & Basavaraju, N. (1991). The prevalence of tardive dyskinesia. *Journal of Clinical Psychopharmacology, 11,* 34-42.

AGITATED BEHAVIOR RATING SCALE (ABRS)

AUTHORS: Donald L. Bliwise and Kathryn A. Lee
ADDRESS: Donald L. Bliwise, PhD, Director
             Emory Sleep Disorders Center
             Emory University School of Medicine
             WMB-Suite 6000, P.O. Drawer V
             Atlanta, GA 30322

DESCRIPTION: The Agitated Behavior Rating Scale (ABRS) was designed by researchers interested in sleep/wake patterns in nursing home residents. It relies on "real time as a key feature in data collection" because "cyclic activity of the central nervous system drives predictable behavioral and physiological events across the 24-hour day" (Bliwise & Lee, 1993, p. 121). The scale, which taps physical and vocal dimensions of agitation, allows observers to record the actual time when agitation occurs. Unlike other agitation scales, which refer to cumulative impressions about agitation and treat agitation as if it were a trait, this instrument structures observations in a real-time framework and allows events surrounding agitation to be studied.

PSYCHOMETRIC PROPERTIES: Content validity for the scale is based on Cohen-Mansfield's conceptual framework (Cohen-Mansfield, 1986; Cohen-Mansfield & Billig, 1986; Cohen-Mansfield, Marx, & Rosenthal, 1989). The authors of the ABRS used items from the Cohen-Mansfield Agitation Inventory (see entry in this book) in the derivation of their two-factor scale. Construct validity of the ABRS was supported in a study showing seasonal changes in agitation, with more agitation during winter (Bliwise, Carroll, Lee, Neckich, & Dement, 1993). To test interrater reliability, 11 nursing home residents were simultaneously and independently observed by three trained raters during rounds on a skilled nursing floor. Residents were rated for physical and vocal agitation during various times of day on five different days. There were 2,745 observations. Percentages of agreement between pairs of raters for presence or absence of agitated behavior ranged between 85.5% and 96.8%, and the percentage of agreement for ratings of intensity was 91.8%.

PROCEDURE: The rater makes discrete observations in a time period lasting 10 to 20 seconds. The scale refers to five areas of behavior: (a) carphologic behavior (i.e, aimless picking and plucking), (b) restraint removal behavior, (c) searching behavior, (d) tapping/banging behavior, and (e) vocalization behavior. For each area, examples for intensity are provided on the scale. Areas (a) through (d) are categorized as physical agitation. Raters designate only one physical agitation behavior during any given observation period. Continuous observations using the method would be possible using video-tape.

SAMPLE ITEM: "A man stands in the dining hall and begins rearranging furniture for no apparent reason" (Bliwise & Lee, 1993, p. 123).

SCORING: Intensity of a behavior is rated as 0 (*not present*), 1 (*low*), 2 (*mild*), or 3 (*high*). Analysis of the data would allow a clinician or researcher to compute for daily, weekly, seasonal, or situational patterns of agitated behavior.

SOURCE: The scale appears in Bliwise and Lee (1993). Reprints of the article are available from the primary author.

REFERENCES

Bliwise, D. L., Carroll, J. S., Lee, K. A., Neckich, J. C., & Dement, W. C. (1993). Sleep and sundowning in nursing home patients with dementia. *Psychiatry Research, 48,* 277-292.

Bliwise, D. L., & Lee, K. A. (1993). Development of an agitated behavior rating scale for discrete temporal observations. *Journal of Nursing Measurement, 1,* 115-124.

Cohen-Mansfield, J. (1986). Agitated behaviors in the elderly: II. Preliminary results in the cognitively deteriorated. *Journal of the American Geriatrics Society, 34,* 722-727.

Cohen-Mansfield, J., & Billig, N. (1986). Agitated behaviors in the elderly: II. A conceptual review. *Journal of the American Geriatrics Society, 34,* 711-721.

Cohen-Mansfield, J., Marx, M. S., & Rosenthal, A. (1989). A description of agitation in a nursing home. *Journal of Gerontology: Medical Sciences, 44*(3), M77-M84.

ALZHEIMER'S DISEASE ASSESSMENT SCALE (ADAS)

AUTHOR: Richard C. Mohs
ADDRESS: Richard C. Mohs, PhD
            Psychiatry Service (116A)
            Mount Sinai School of Medicine
            VA Medical Center
            130 West Kingsbridge Road
            Bronx, NY 10468

DESCRIPTION: The Alzheimer's Disease Assessment Scale (ADAS) is an instrument used to rate severity of dysfunction in all of the "cognitive and noncognitive behaviors characteristic of persons with Alzheimer's Disease" (Rosen, Mohs, & Davis, 1984, p. 1359). There are two subscales: cognitive and noncognitive. The two can be used separately or together (Mohs, 1994). The cognitive portion includes items for memory, attention, orientation, language, and praxis. The noncognitive portion, applicable to some Alzheimer's disease (AD) patients, includes mood, agitation, and psychotic features. The ADAS was designed to be used in studies of the effects of drugs on the cognition or behavioral impairments of AD. It is also appropriate for longitudinal studies (Stern et al., 1994) and as a measure for evaluating caregiving environments (Swanson, Maas, & Buckwalter, 1994). Severely demented patients cannot be assessed with the ADAS.

PSYCHOMETRIC PROPERTIES: Rosen et al. (1984) developed the original ADAS using samples of AD patients ($n = 27$) and normal controls ($n = 28$). Two raters independently evaluated each subject with the ADAS, and 1 to 2 months later, 44 subjects were reevaluated. Initially, the ADAS had 40 items; after testing, the authors adopted a 21-item version that included only those items with significant interrater and test-retest reliability. Validity was supported by correlations of ADAS scores with scores on the Blessed Dementia Scale and Information-Memory-Concentration Test (see entry in this book). In a study of residents of a special care unit ($N = 22$), Swanson et al. (1994) found correlations ranging from 0.88 to 0.91 for scores on the ADAS with other measures of deterioration. They also demonstrated internal consistency (0.84 to 0.94) and interrater reliability (0.70 to 0.79) for the ADAS. In a longitudinal study of 111 AD patients and 72 normal elders, Stern et al. (1994) showed that the cognitive subscale of the ADAS was sensitive to changes in both mild and severe dementia (p. 390).

PROCEDURE: Administration of the ADAS requires preparation. There are very specific rules for administration (Mohs, 1994). The ADAS has clinician-rated items as well as items to elicit performance. The subject is interviewed and also completes cognitive tasks. Information to complete the noncognitive portion of the test is gathered from the subject and a knowledgeable informant. Completion takes approximately 45 minutes (Mohs, 1995, p. 1381). When the ADAS is administered to the same individual more than once, alternate forms are used for the word recall and word recognition items (Mohs, 1994).

SAMPLE ITEM:

Orientation: The components of orientation are date, month, year, day of the week, season, time of day, place, and person. The tester should ask the patient for these pieces of information one at a time. Before giving this item, the tester should be sure that no clocks, watches or calendars are visible to aid the patient.

One point is given for each incorrect response (maximum = 8). Acceptable answers include + or −1 for the date; within 1 hour for the hour; partial name for place; naming of upcoming season within one week before its onset, and name of previous season for two weeks after its termination. Month, year, day of the week and the person's first and last name must be exact. (Mohs, 1994, p. 7)

SCORING: The rating scale for each item ranges from 0 for *no impairment,* or absence of a behavior, to 5 for *severe impairment,* or very high frequency of a behavior. The other ratings—1, 2, 3, and 4—are assigned for very mild, mild, moderate, and moderately severe assessments. Scores for the cognitive component of the scale range between 0, indicating no impairment, and 75, indicating severe impairment (Mohs, 1994, p. 1). The noncognitive component has seven clinician-rated items.

SOURCE: The original scale was printed as an appendix to Rosen et al. (1984). However, there have been some changes in the format, order, and scoring since 1984. The most recent version of the instrument is in Mohs (1994), which is available from the author. The Mount Sinai School of Medicine owns the copyright to the 1994 version of the instrument.

REFERENCES

Mohs, R. C. (1994). *Administration and scoring manual for the Alzheimer's Disease Assessment Scale.* (Available from the author at address listed above)

Mohs, R. C. (1995). Neuropsychological assessment of patients with Alzheimer's disease. In F. E. Bloom & D. J. Kupfer (Eds.), *Psychopharmacology: The fourth generation of progress* (pp. 1377-1388). New York: Raven.

Rosen, W. G., Mohs, R. C., & Davis, K. L. (1984). A new rating scale for Alzheimer's disease. *American Journal of Psychiatry, 141,* 1356-1364.

Stern, R. G., Mohs, R. C., Davidson, M., Schmeidler, J., Silverman, J., Kramer-Ginsberg, E., Searcey, T., Bierer, L., & Davis, K. L. (1994). A longitudinal study of Alzheimer's disease: Measurement, rate, and predictors of cognitive deterioration. *American Journal of Psychiatry, 151,* 390-396.

Swanson, E. A., Maas, M. L., & Buckwalter, K. C. (1994). Alzheimer's residents' cognitive and functional measures: Special and traditional care unit comparison. *Clinical Nursing Research, 3,* 27-41.

ANXIETY STATUS INVENTORY (ASI) AND SELF-RATING ANXIETY SCALE (SAS)

AUTHOR: William W. K. Zung
ADDRESS: Elizabeth Marsh Zung
           1816 Woodburn Road
           Durham, NC 27705

DESCRIPTION: The Anxiety Status Inventory (ASI) is a 20-item scale designed to measure anxiety as a clinical disorder rather than as a trait or a feeling state (Zung, 1971). The ASI is completed by a clinician who makes judgments about the presence and extent of symptoms based on clinical observations and information provided by the patient in an interview. When a symptom is present, the clinician-interviewer inquires further about its severity, asking about intensity, duration, and frequency. The Self-Rating Anxiety Scale (SAS), the companion instrument to the ASI, also has 20 items. SAS items are phrased as subjective statements about the same symptoms detailed in the ASI. Some items are phrased symptomatically positive and some negative "so that the patient is less able to discern a trend in the answers" (p. 375). On both scales, there are 5 items for "affective" symptoms and 15 items related to "somatic" symptoms (p. 371).

PSYCHOMETRIC PROPERTIES: Zung derived the items for the tools from experience and review of the literature. He administered the SAS and another measure of anxiety, the Taylor Manifest Anxiety Scale, to 152 inpatients and 73 outpatients of a psychiatric service. The mean age was 41, with a range from 14 to 75. Fifty of the outpatients were women. All inpatients were men. The patients were later interviewed, and the ASI was completed. Each patient was also diagnosed by a psychiatrist who was blind to anxiety ratings. ASIs were analyzed for five diagnostic groups. One hundred "normal" controls also completed the SAS. Results showed that ASI scores differentiated patients with anxiety disorders; their scores were significantly higher than those of any other group (Zung, 1971, p. 377). Mean SAS scores for the normal controls were lower than mean scores for all five patient groups. The correlation between ASI and SAS scores was 0.74. Split-half reliability correlations (even/odd) for the ASI and SAS were 0.83 and 0.71 respectively (p. 378).

PROCEDURE: Observers use the prescribed interview guide with the ASI to ensure that all areas of the inventory are covered. The author stressed the need, however, for flexibility in asking questions so that the patient experiences a "smooth interview that does not sound like a question-answer examination" (Zung, 1976a, p. 200). Zung (1971) outlined several specific rules for making ratings (pp. 372-375). There is a standard time context of 1 week for both instruments. Zung (1976a) recommended that some questions for the ASI be prefaced with the phrase "During the past week, have you . . . ?" (p. 200). Sheikh (1991) pointed out that ASI interviewers must be cautious when dealing with the 1-week time context because some ASI items begin with the phrase "Do you ever . . . ?"

SAMPLE ASI ITEMS:

Affective and Somatic Symptoms of Anxiety	Interview Guide
1. Anxiousness	1. Do you ever feel nervous and anxious?
9. Restlessness	9. Do you find yourself restless and can't sit still?
20. Nightmares	20. Do you have dreams that scare you?

(Zung, 1971, p. 373)

CORRESPONDING SAS ITEMS:

Affective and Somatic Symptoms of Anxiety	Self-Rating Form
1. Anxiousness	1. I feel more nervous and anxious than usual.
9. Restlessness	9. I feel calm and sit still easily.
20. Nightmares	20. I have nightmares.

(Zung, 1976b, p. 338)

SCORING: ASI items are rated on a 4-point scale: *none* (1), *mild* (2), *moderate* (3), and *severe* (4). SAS items are rated *none or a little of the time* (1), *some of the time* (2), *a good part of the time* (3), or *most or all of the time* (4). Total ASI or SAS raw scores are the sums of item ratings. A Z score for the ASI can be derived by dividing the total raw score by the maximum possible score of 80 and multiplying by 100 (Zung, 1971, p. 376). The same calculations can be applied to convert SAS scores to what Zung termed the SAS "index" (pp. 376-377).

SOURCE: The ASI and its counterpart, the SAS, are reprinted in Zung (1971). They also appear in Zung (1976a, 1976b). Elizabeth Marsh Zung, who owns the copyright to her late husband's instruments, may be contacted by those needing permission to use them.

REFERENCES

Sheikh, J. I. (1991). Anxiety rating scales for the elderly. In C. Salzman & B. D. Lebowitz (Eds.), *Anxiety in the elderly: Treatment and research* (pp. 251-265). New York: Springer.

Zung, W. W. K. (1971). A rating instrument for anxiety disorders. *Psychosomatics, 12,* 371-379.

Zung, W. W. K. (1976a). Anxiety Status Inventory. In W. Guy (Ed.), *Early Clinical Drug Evaluation Unit assessment manual for psychopharmacology* (Rev. ed., pp. 200-204, DHEW Pub. No. ADM 76-338). Washington, DC: U.S. Department of Health, Education and Welfare.

Zung, W. W. K. (1976b). SAS. In W. Guy (Ed.), *Early Clinical Drug Evaluation Unit assessment manual for psychopharmacology* (Rev. ed., pp. 338-340, DHEW Pub. No. ADM 76-338). Washington, DC: U.S. Department of Health, Education and Welfare.

ARTHRITIS IMPACT MEASUREMENT SCALES—REVISED (AIMS2)

AUTHORS: Robert F. Meenan, Paul M. Gertman, and John H. Mason
ADDRESS: Robert F. Meenan, MD
            Boston University School of Medicine
            The Arthritis Center
            80 East Concord Street
            Boston, MA 02118-2394

DESCRIPTION: The Arthritis Impact Measurement Scales (AIMS2) are a revised version of the initial AIMS, "an improvement on an evaluation instrument that was developed to measure patient outcomes in the rheumatic diseases" (Meenan & Mason, 1994, p. 1). The AIMS2 is a 78-item questionnaire with 12 scales designed to measure health status, conceived as a multidimensional construct of physical, mental, and social well-being (Meenan, Gertman, & Mason, 1980). The scales refer to "mobility level, walking and bending, hand and finger function, arm function, self-care tasks, household tasks, social activity, support from family and friends, arthritis pain, work, level of tension, and mood" (Meenan & Mason, 1994, p. 1).

PSYCHOMETRIC PROPERTIES: Validity, reliability, and sensitivity for the AIMS2 were established in work with the initial version of the AIMS. For the original questionnaire, the authors adopted items from other established instruments, adding new arthritis-specific and clinically relevant scales (Meenan et al., 1980, p. 147). One hundred and four arthritis patients partici-pated in a pilot study. Following revisions, the AIMS was tested again with a national sample ($N = 625$) of arthritis patients who had an average age of 53 years (78% younger than 65 years), an average education of 12 years, and an average income between $10,000 and $15,000 (Meenan, Gertman, Mason, & Dunaif, 1982). AIMS scores correlated well with estimates of functional status made by physicians and with brief clinical status assessments ($N = 100$). Alpha coefficients for the scales exceeded 0.7; test-retest correlations exceeded 0.8 (p. 1049). Mason, Weener, Gertman, and Meenan (1983) showed that the AIMS could be used to measure health status in individuals with chronic diseases other than arthritis. AIMS scores of chronically ill individuals (mean age = 60; $N = 84$) with diabetes, ostomies, osteoarthritis, and rheumatoid arthritis have been shown to be stable over a 6-week period (Burckhardt, Woods, Schultz, & Ziebarth, 1989). Comparison of the AIMS with a similar and independently developed measure, the Health Assessment Questionnaire (HAQ), demonstrated that the two instruments, though differ-ent, "measured similar dimensions of health status" (Brown et al., 1984, p. 160); AIMS scores were highly correlated with scores on the HAQ (0.91).

PROCEDURE: The AIMS2 was designed to be self-administered. Respon-dents should not be coached; rather, they should merely be given the ques-tionnaire and asked to complete it. It takes about 20 minutes to complete the AIMS2.

SAMPLE ITEMS: "During the past month, did you need help to take a bath or shower?" and "During the past month, how often did your morning stiffness last more than one hour from the time you woke up?" (Meenan, Gertman, & Mason, 1990).

SCORING: Low values on the AIMS2 are associated with high health status. Some items are written to avoid response bias and require reverse coding. The *AIMS2 User's Guide* (Meenan & Mason, 1994) provides coding infor-mation and procedures for "normalization" of scores so that they can "be expressed in the range 0-10" (p. 2). The guide also includes instructions for adjusting AIMS2 scores for comorbidity and for use with samples over age 60.

SOURCE: The *AIMS2 User's Guide* (Meenan & Mason, 1994) and the instrument are available from the authors at the Boston University Arthritis Center. The staff of the center will "assist users with application strategies and data processing" (Meenan & Mason, 1994, p. 3). The copyright for the AIMS2 is owned by Boston University. Researchers or clinicians who want to use the AIMS2 need permission from the authors.

REFERENCES

Brown, J. H., Kazis, L. E., Spitz, P. W., Gertman, P., Fries, J. F., & Meenan, R. F. (1984). The dimensions of health outcomes: A cross-validated examination of health status measurement. *American Journal of Public Health, 74,* 159-161.

Burckhardt, C. S., Woods, S. L., Schultz, A. A., & Ziebarth, D. M. (1989). Quality of life of adults with chronic illness: A psychometric study. *Research in Nursing and Health, 12,* 347-354.

Mason, J. H., Weener, J. L., Gertman, P. M., & Meenan, R. F. (1983). Health status in chronic disease: A comparative study of rheumatoid arthritis. *Journal of Rheumatology, 10,* 763-768.

Meenan, R. F., Gertman, P. M., & Mason, J. H. (1980). Measuring health status in arthritis. *Arthritis and Rheumatism, 23,* 146-152.

Meenan, R. F., Gertman, P. M., & Mason, J. H. (1990). *Arthritis Impact Measurement Scales—Revised.* (Available from the authors at address listed above)

Meenan, R. F., Gertman, P. M., Mason, J. H., & Dunaif, R. (1982). The Arthritis Impact Measurement Scales: Further investigation of a health status instrument. *Arthritis and Rheumatism, 25,* 1048-1053.

Meenan, R. F., & Mason, J. H. (1994). *AIMS2 user's guide.* (Available from the authors at address listed above)

BARTHEL INDEX (BI)

AUTHORS: Dorothea W. Barthel and Florence Mahoney

DESCRIPTION: The Barthel Index was developed in the 1950s as a "simple index of independence to score the ability of a patient with a neuromuscular or musculoskeletal disorder to care for himself, and by repeating the test periodically, to assess his improvement" (Mahoney & Barthel, 1965, p. 61). It has been used extensively in long-term care and rehabilitation settings. Before it was initially published, its validity had been established in 10 years of work with patients in chronic disease hospitals (Mahoney, Wood, & Barthel, 1958). Items refer to (a) feeding, (b) moving from wheelchair to bed and return, (c) doing personal toilet, (d) getting on and off toilet, (e) bathing self, (f) walking on a level surface, (g) propelling a wheelchair, (h) ascending and descending stairs, (i) dressing and undressing, (j) continence of bowels, and (k) continence of bladder. The weights for score (0, 5, 10, or 15) were "based on the time and amount of actual physical assistance required if a patient is unable to perform the activity" (Mahoney & Barthel, 1965, p. 61). Incontinence, for example, was weighted heavily because it required so much time from caregivers.

PSYCHOMETRIC PROPERTIES: Validity of the BI was studied prospectively with 486 rehabilitation patients. Stroke patients "with low scores had a higher subsequent mortality than those with high scores," and "the greater the rise in score while in hospital, the more likely was the patient to be classified as clinically improved" (Wylie & White, 1964, p. 837). An expanded, scaled version of the index, called the Barthel Self-Care Ratings, was studied by Granger, Albrecht, and Hamilton (1979). Kane and Kane (1981) cited Lawton's view that the original Barthel scale is most appropriate for rehabilitation clients, whereas the "Likert self-care scales are a better measure for geriatric patients" (p. 49). Kane and Kane (1981) also cited Sherwood's data for internal consistency of the Barthel Self-Care Ratings, alpha coefficients ranging between 0.953 and 0.965 (p. 49). The reliability of the instrument, in another format, was studied by Collin, Wade, Davies, and Horne (1988). Twenty-five stroke and head injury patients, ranging in age from 12 to over 65, were independently rated on the BI in four different ways. The coefficient of concordance between the four ratings (0.93, $p < 0.001$) was high and significant (p. 61). Collin et al. (1988) and Wade and Collin (1988) suggested that the BI be adopted as a standard measure for rehabilitation settings.

PROCEDURE: When using the original index, the observer follows very specific guidelines to assign a score—0, 5, 10, or 15, depending on the item—for each of 11 activities. The authors noted that the BI "can easily be understood by all who work with a patient and can accurately and quickly be scored by anyone who adheres to the definitions of items" (Mahoney & Barthel, 1965, p. 65).

SAMPLE ITEM: "Bathing Self. 5 = Patient may use a bath tub, a shower, or take a complete sponge bath. He must be able to do all steps involved in whichever method is employed without another person being present" (Mahoney & Barthel, 1965, p. 63). Note: For the "Bathing Self" item, 5 and 0 are the only possible scores. The patient scores 0 if even minimal help is required.

SCORING: The range of scores is between 0 and 100.

SOURCE: The instrument and its original scoring guidelines are available in Mahoney and Barthel (1965) and Wylie and White (1964). The instrument is also available in the modified format suggested by Collin et al. (1988) and the version adopted by Granger et al. (1979) for rehabilitation settings.

REFERENCES

Collin, C., Wade, D. T., Davies, S., & Horne, V. (1988). Barthel ADL Index: A reliability study. *International Disability Studies, 10,* 61-63.

Granger, C. V., Albrecht, G. L., & Hamilton, B. B. (1979). Outcome of comprehensive medical rehabilitation: Measurement by PULSES Profile and the Barthel Index. *Archives of Physical Medicine and Rehabilitation, 60,* 145-154.

Kane, R. A., & Kane, R. L. (1981). *Assessing the elderly: A practical guide to measurement.* Lexington, MA: D. C. Heath.

Mahoney, F. I., & Barthel, D. W. (1965). Functional evaluation: The Barthel Index. *Maryland State Medical Journal, 14*(2), 61-65.

Mahoney, F. I., Wood, O. H., & Barthel, D. W. (1958). Rehabilitation of chronically ill patients. *Southern Medical Journal, 51,* 605-609.

Wade, D. T., & Collin, C. (1988). The Barthel ADL index: A standard measure of physical disability? *International Disability Studies, 10,* 64-67.

Wylie, C. M., & White, B. K. (1964). A measure of disability. *Archives of Environmental Health, 8,* 834-839.

BECK DEPRESSION INVENTORY (BDI)

AUTHORS: Aaron T. Beck and Associates
ADDRESS: The Psychological Corporation
             555 Academic Court
             San Antonio, TX 78204-0952

DESCRIPTION: This widely used instrument was designed to measure behavioral manifestations of depression and to arrive at a quantitative assessment of the intensity of depression. Items were derived from 21 clinically observed categories of symptoms and attitudes. They include mood, pessimism, sense of failure, lack of satisfaction, guilty feeling, sense of punishment, self-hate, self-accusation, self-punitive wishes, crying spells, irritability, social withdrawal, indecisiveness, body image, work inhibition, sleep disturbance, fatigability, loss of appetite, weight loss, somatic preoccupation, and loss of libido. For each category, there is a series of four self-evaluative statements, ranked to reflect a range of severity. There are both long (21 categories) and short (13 categories) forms of the BDI. It has been translated into many languages.

PSYCHOMETRIC PROPERTIES: The inventory, which has been used in more than 600 studies (Shaver & Brennan, 1991), initially was administered to a random sample of 226 psychiatric patients and another "replication" group of 183. The sample was predominantly Caucasian and had a high frequency of persons from lower socioeconomic groups. Ages ranged between 15 and 55+, with the greatest concentration between 15 and 44. Internal consistency has been demonstrated with high correlations for split-half analysis and between scores for all 21 categories and total scores. Independent clinical ratings of the depth of depression, made by experienced psychiatrists, correlate with BDI scores (0.65 and 0.67, $p < 0.01$). In a group of 38 patients, the BDI was sensitive to change after 2 to 5 weeks. Construct validity was demonstrated in five different studies in which the test was used as a criterion measure (Beck & Beamesderfer, 1974, p. 159). Factor analyses "generally reveal three intercorrelated factors: negative attitudes or suicide, physiological, and performance difficulty" (Shaver & Brennan, 1991, p. 202).

PROCEDURE: The inventory can be administered by an interviewer who reads each statement aloud to the patient, who also has a copy. The interviewer asks the patient to choose the statement that currently fits him or her best. The BDI may also be completed as a self-report. Gallagher (1986) urged four areas of caution about using the BDI with the elderly: (a) An eighth-grade reading level is needed to comprehend the tool, (b) both under- and overreporting of symptoms has been found in the elder population, (c) somatic complaints may not be true indicators of depression in this age group, and (d) cognitively impaired elders have difficulty with this scale.

SAMPLE ITEM:

0	I don't feel that I am any worse than anybody else.
1	I am critical of myself for weaknesses or mistakes.
2	I blame myself for my faults.
3	I blame myself for everything bad that happens.

(Beck, Ward, Mendelson, Mock, & Erbaugh, 1961, p. 570)

SCORING: The BDI yields a single score obtained by adding the scores for the individual categories. Values from 0 to 3 are assigned to statements from which the respondent chooses; therefore, scores may range from 0 to 63. According to the authors (Beck & Beamesderfer, 1974, p. 159), there should be no arbitrary cutoff scores. Rather, the clinician or researcher should choose a cutoff based on the population and the purposes for which the BDI is being used. The following norms, however, have been reported as "used conventionally": "0-9 normal range; 10-15 mild depression; 16-19 mild to moderate depression; 20-29 moderate to severe depression; 30-63 severe depression" (Gallagher, 1986, p. 151). Stewart et al. (1991) administered the BDI to 1,048 elders in Florida and found that 13.7% of the men and 20.6% of the women scored above 10. Women and individuals with lower educational attainment tend to score higher (more depressed) on the BDI.

SOURCE: The tool is available from the Psychological Corporation. The initial version of the tool appears in the appendix to Beck et al. (1961). The short form is in the appendix to Beck and Beamesderfer (1974).

REFERENCES

Beck, A. T., & Beamesderfer, A. (1974). Assessment of depression: The depression inventory. In *Modern Problems in Pharmacopsychiatry: Vol. 7. Psychological Measurement in Psychopharmacology* (pp. 151-169). Basel, Switzerland: Karger.

Beck, A. T., Ward, C. H., Mendelson, M., Mock, J., & Erbaugh, J. (1961). An inventory for measuring depression. *Archives of General Psychiatry, 4,* 561-571.

Gallagher, D. (1986). The Beck Depression Inventory and older adults. *Clinical Gerontologist, 5,* 149-163.

Shaver, P. R., & Brennan, K. A. (1991). Measures of depression and loneliness. In J. P. Robinson, P. R. Shaver, & L. S. Wrightsman (Eds.), *Measures of personality and social psychological attitudes* (pp. 195-289). San Diego: Academic Press.

Stewart, R. B., Blashfield, R., Hale, W. E., Moore, M. T., May, F. E., & Marks, R. G. (1991). Correlates of Beck Depression Inventory scores in an ambulatory elderly population: Symptoms, diseases, laboratory values, and medications. *Journal of Family Practice, 32,* 497-502.

BECK HOPELESSNESS SCALE (BHS)

AUTHORS: Aaron T. Beck and Associates
ADDRESS: The Psychological Corporation
            555 Academic Court
            San Antonio, TX 78204-0952

DESCRIPTION: Construction of the Beck Hopelessness Scale (BHS) was based on the assumption "that hopelessness can readily be objectified by defining it as a system of cognitive schemas whose common denomination is negative expectations about the future" (Beck, Weissman, Lester, & Trexler, 1974, p. 864). The scale is a self-report instrument with a 20-item true-false format. Items for the BHS were drawn both from "a test of attitudes about the future" and "from a pool of pessimistic statements made by psychiatric patients who were adjudged by clinicians to appear hopeless" (p. 861).

PSYCHOMETRIC PROPERTIES: The BHS was piloted with groups of depressed and nondepressed patients and with clinicians, who were asked to give opinions about the content and clarity of item language. Following revisions of wording, the scale was tested for internal consistency (0.93) with a group of middle-aged patients ($N = 294$) who had attempted suicide. Item-to-total score correlations ranged from 0.39 to 0.76 (p. 863). Factor analyses of data from this sample tapped "affective, motivational and cognitive" aspects of hopelessness. Factors were labeled "Feelings About the Future," "Loss of Motivation," and "Future Expectations" (Beck et al., 1974, p. 864). To estimate concurrent validity, Beck et al. correlated clinicians' global ratings of hopelessness with BHS scores for a sample of 23 general medical practice outpatients (0.74; $p < 0.001$) and 62 hospitalized suicidal patients (0.62; $p < 0.001$). Further support for concurrent validity was demonstrated when scores of 59 depressed hospitalized patients on the BHS were significantly correlated with their scores on a semantic differential test about the future (0.60; $p < 0.001$), and with the pessimism item of the Beck Depression Inventory (see entry in this book; 0.63; $p < 0.001$). These tests were repeated with the 59 patients at the time of their discharge. All scores were reduced, and the changes in scores were correlated (0.49; $p < 0.01$). Construct validity for the BHS was supported in four studies related to negative expectancies and depression (Beck et al., 1974, p. 863).

Following on the work of others that they cited, Farran, Salloway, and Clark (1990) adapted all 20 items from the BHS and used them to test hope in a sample of community-dwelling elderly. The adapted scale, which has a Likert format, is called the Hopefulness Scale (HS). Farran et al. reported a different factor structure and presented arguments about conceptual changes needed when measuring hope or hopelessness in the elderly.

PROCEDURE: The BHS is presented in a paper-and-pencil format. The respondent answers "true" or "false" to 20 items.

SAMPLE ITEMS: "I might as well give up because I can't make things better for myself" and "When things are going badly, I am helped by knowing they can't stay that way forever" (Beck et al., 1974, p. 862).

SCORING: Nine items are designed to be considered false by a hopeless person, and 11 are designed to be considered true. The score assigned to each item is 0 (*not hopeless*) or 1 (*hopeless*). The sum of item scores is the hopelessness score. Scores range between 0 and 20.

SOURCE: The tool is available from the Psychological Corporation. Items for the scale are reprinted in Beck et al. (1974).

REFERENCES

Beck, A. T., Weissman, A., Lester, D., & Trexler, L. (1974). The measurement of pessimism: The hopelessness scale. *Journal of Consulting and Clinical Psychology, 42,* 861-865.
Farran, C. J., Salloway, J. C., & Clark, D. C. (1990). Measurement of hope in a community-based older population. *Western Journal of Nursing Research, 12,* 42-59.

BEDFORD ALZHEIMER NURSING SEVERITY SCALE (BANS-S)

AUTHORS: Ladislav Volicer, Ann C. Hurley, and colleagues
ADDRESS: Ladislav Volicer, MD, PhD
            Geriatric Research, Education and Clinical Center
            Edith Nourse Rogers Memorial Veterans Hospital
            200 Springs Road
            Bedford, MA 01730

DESCRIPTION: The Bedford Alzheimer Nursing Severity Scale (BANS-S) is a seven-item modification of an earlier eight-item instrument (Volicer et al., 1987). Ratings of cognition, functional deficits, and pathological symptoms, such as disturbance of sleep-wake cycle and muscle rigidity, are combined in this scale, which is sensitive even for severely impaired persons. The seven areas of assessment addressed by the BANS-S are dressing, sleeping, speech, eating, mobility, muscles, and eye contact.

PSYCHOMETRIC PROPERTIES: Content validity was evaluated by expert geriatric nurses with clinical experience in dementia special care units. The instrument was tested with a sample of 74 geropsychiatric patients. Mean age was 72.4; 71 patients were males and 3 were females; 73 were Caucasian. Alpha coefficients ranged from 0.64 to 0.80. BANS-S scores were significantly correlated with other measures of activities of daily living, language assessment, and mental status. BANS-S scores showed greater sensitivity over time. Compared with scores on other instruments, which were not sensitive once speech was lost, there were significant changes in BANS-S scores during a 3-month period.

PROCEDURE: Ratings are completed by a person familiar with and/or informed about the subject's behaviors on a 24-hour basis.

SAMPLE ITEM: Eating.

1. Eats independently
2. Requires minimal assistance and/or coaxing
3. Requires moderate assistance and/or coaxing
4. Completely dependent (Volicer, Hurley, Lathi, & Kowall, 1994, p. M226)

SCORING: The range of scores is from 7 (*no impairment*) to 28 (*complete impairment*).

SOURCE: A copy of the scale appears in Volicer et al. (1994).

REFERENCES

Volicer, L., Hurley, A. C., Lathi, D. C., & Kowall, N. W. (1994). Measurement of severity in advanced Alzheimer's disease. *Journal of Gerontology: Medical Sciences, 49,* M223-M226.

Volicer, L., Selter, B., Rheaume, Y., Fabiszewski, K., Herz, L., Shapiro, R., & Innis, P. (1987). Progression of Alzheimer-type dementia in institutionalized patients: A cross-sectional study. *Journal of Applied Gerontology, 6,* 83-94.

BERG BALANCE SCALE (BBS)

AUTHOR: Katherine Berg
ADDRESS: Katherine Berg, PhD, PT
            Brown University
            Center for Gerontology and Health Care Research
            Box G-B222
            Providence, RI 02912

DESCRIPTION: The Berg Balance Scale (BBS) is an instrument designed for use in rehabilitation and geriatric settings where clinical or research goals would include measuring postural control and preventing falls. The BBS tests "the ability of an individual to maintain balance while performing 14 movements required in everyday living" (Berg, Wood-Dauphinee, Williams, & Maki, 1992, p. S7).

PSYCHOMETRIC PROPERTIES: Content validity for the instrument was supported by the evaluations of health care professionals and elderly persons who took part in a preliminary study of the instrument. Validity and reliability of the scale were estimated in studies with samples of nursing home residents ($n = 113$), acute care stroke patients ($n = 70$), and elderly subjects who submitted to laboratory testing ($n = 31$). Reliability of the scale was demonstrated with intraclass correlations for interrater (0.92 to 0.98) and intrarater (0.91 to 0.99) comparisons. Alphas for the scale ranged between 0.83 and 0.97 (Berg, Wood-Dauphinee, & Williams, 1995). Scores on the BBS discriminated between nursing home residents subgrouped by use of walking devices. Balance scores for this sample were correlated with global ratings for balance made by caregivers (0.47 to 0.61) and by participants themselves (0.39 to 0.41). Balance scores were also significant predictors of falls (Berg et al., 1992, pp. S8-S9). BBS scores of stroke patients were correlated with scores on the Barthel Index (see entry in this book; 0.80) and another measure of physical performance (0.62 to 0.94). BBS scores distinguished between patients grouped by follow-up status; patients were either at home (45.0), in rehabilitation centers (31.1), or still in the hospital (8.6). For the sample tested in the laboratory, correlations between BBS scores and scores on another balance index (0.91), the Timed "Up and Go" Test (see entry in this book; 0.76), and the mobility score of the Barthel Index (0.67) supported the validity of the BBS (p. S10).

PROCEDURE: The examiner provides instructions for each item, exactly as they are printed on the BBS form. Each mobility task is actually demonstrated for the examiner by the subject.

SAMPLE ITEM: Standing on One Leg.

Instructions: Stand on one leg as long as you can without holding.	
4	Able to lift leg independently and hold > 10 seconds
3	Able to lift leg independently and hold 5-10 seconds
2	Able to lift leg independently and hold = or > 3 seconds
1	Tries to lift leg unable to hold 3 seconds but remains standing independently
0	Unable to try or needs assist to prevent fall

(Berg, 1988, p. 4)

SCORING: Scores on the BBS range from 0 to 56 points. Berg et al. (1992) considered a score of 45 to be the "cut-off point between those individuals who are safe in independent ambulation and those requiring investigation concerning need for assistive devices or supervision" (p. S8).

SOURCE: Copies of the BBS are available from the author, who holds a copyright. The scale is also reproduced in Shumway-Cook and Woollacott (1995, pp. 448-451).

REFERENCES

Berg, K. (1988). *Measuring balance in the elderly: Development and validation of an instrument.* Unpublished master's thesis, McGill University. (Available from the author at address listed above)

Berg, K., Wood-Dauphinee, S., & Williams, J. I. (1995). The Balance Scale: Reliability assessment with elderly residents and patients with an acute stroke. *Scandinavian Journal of Rehabilitation Medicine, 27,* 27-36.

Berg, K. O., Wood-Dauphinee, S., Williams, J. I., & Maki, B. (1992). Measuring balance in the elderly: Validation of an instrument. *Canadian Journal of Public Health, 83*(Suppl. 2), S7-S11.

Shumway-Cook, A., & Woollacott, M. (1995). *Motor control: Theory and applications.* Baltimore: Williams & Wilkins.

BLESSED DEMENTIA SCALE (DS) AND INFORMATION-MEMORY-CONCENTRATION TEST (IMC)

AUTHORS: G. Blessed, B. E. Tomlinson, and Sir Martin Roth
ADDRESS: G. Blessed, MB, BS, MRCPE, DPM
            Newcastle General Hospital
            MRC, Neurochemical Pathology Unit
            Newcastle Upon Tyne NE4 6BE, England

DESCRIPTION: The Blessed Dementia Scale (DS) is a 22-item scale for evaluation of changes in the performance of everyday activities, self-care habits, personality, interests, and drives. The DS and its 30-item companion test, the Information-Memory-Concentration test (IMC), were used by Blessed, Tomlinson, and Roth (1968) to quantify "degree of intellectual and personality deterioration" (p. 799) in a study comparing functional and emotional change with underlying brain neuropathology. The scale and test have been widely used with the elderly clinically and have served as standards with which similar tools are compared when initially developed. The DS and IMC have been adopted as components of larger test batteries (Morris, Mohs, Rogers, Fillenbaum, & Heyman, 1988), combined with other instruments for more comprehensive assessments (Weiler, Chiroboga, & Black, 1994), and revised into shorter formats (Katzman et al., 1983; Kay, 1977).

PSYCHOMETRIC PROPERTIES: Blessed et al. (1968) demonstrated that scores for these instruments were related to the counts of senile plaques in the brains of 60 patients such that there was a "tendency for functional incapacity to increase as mean plaque count increased" and "a tendency for performance on the test to decline with increasing plaque formation" (pp. 802-803). Erkinjuntti, Hokkanen, Sulkava, and Palo (1988) showed that the DS and its shortened 11-item version (RDS; Kay, 1977) had satisfactory levels of sensitivity and specificity. Villardita and Lomeo (1992) demonstrated test-retest reliability coefficients, 0.88 for the DS and 0.89 for the IMC.

PROCEDURE: The respondent to the DS is "a close relative or friend" who answers questions about the patient's "competence in personal, domestic and social activities . . . during the preceding six months" (Blessed et al., 1968,

p. 799). Patients themselves respond to the IMC, which measures "orientation, remote memory, recent memory, and concentration" (p. 799).

SAMPLE DS ITEM: "Inability to interpret surroundings (e.g., to recognize whether in hospital, or at home, to discriminate between patients, doctors and nurses, relatives and hospital staff, etc.)" (Blessed et al., 1968, p. 808).

SAMPLE IMC ITEMS: "Date of World War I" and "Counting 20 to 1" (Blessed et al., 1968, p. 809).

SCORING: For the DS, the highest score (28) indicates "extreme incapacity." A score of 0 shows "fully preserved capacity." For the IMC, the direction of scoring is reversed, with 0 indicating "complete failure" and the highest score (37) "representing full marks in the complete battery" (Blessed et al., 1968, p. 799).

SOURCE: The instruments and scoring rules appear in the appendix to Blessed et al. (1968) and are copyrighted by the *British Journal of Psychiatry.* They have also been reprinted in Blessed, Tomlinson, and Roth (1988).

REFERENCES

Blessed, G., Tomlinson, B. E., & Roth, M. (1968). The association between quantitative measures of dementia and senile changes in the cerebral gray matter of elderly subjects. *British Journal of Psychiatry, 114,* 797-811.

Blessed, G., Tomlinson, B. E., & Roth, M. (1988). Blessed-Roth Dementia Scale. *Psychopharmacology Bulletin, 24,* 706-708.

Erkinjuntti, T., Hokkanen, L., Sulkava, R., & Palo, J. (1988). The Blessed Dementia Scale as a screening test for dementia. *International Journal of Geriatric Psychiatry, 3,* 267-273.

Katzman, R., Brown, T., Fuld, P., Peck, A., Schecter, R., & Schimmel, H. (1983). Validation of a short orientation-memory-concentration test of cognitive impairment. *American Journal of Psychiatry, 140,* 734-739.

Kay, D. W. K. (1977). Epidemiology and identification of brain deficit in the elderly. In C. Eisdorfer & R. O. Friedel (Eds.), *Cognitive and emotional disturbance in the elderly: Clinical issues* (pp. 11-26). Chicago: Year Book Medical Publishers.

Morris, J. C., Mohs, R. C., Rogers, H., Fillenbaum, G., & Heyman, A. (1988). Consortium to Establish a Registry for Alzheimer's Disease (CERAD) clinical and neuropsychological assessment of Alzheimer's disease. *Psychopharmacology Bulletin, 24,* 641-652.

Villardita, C., & Lomeo, C. (1992). Alzheimer's disease: Correlational analysis of three screening tests and three behavioural scales. *Acta Neurologica Scandinavica, 86,* 603-608.

Weiler, P. G., Chiroboga, D. A., & Black, S. A. (1994). Comparison of mental status tests: Implications for Alzheimer's patients and their caregivers. *Journal of Gerontology: Social Sciences, 49,* S44-S51.

BODY CATHEXIS SCALE (BC-SC)

AUTHORS: Paul F. Secord and Sidney M. Jourard

DESCRIPTION: The authors of the Body Cathexis Scale (BC-SC) defined body cathexis as "the degree of feeling of satisfaction or dissatisfaction with the various parts or processes of the body" (Secord & Jourard, 1953, p. 343). They believed that "the individual's attitudes toward his body are of crucial importance to any comprehensive theory of personality" and that body cathexis is "integrally related to the self-concept, although identifiable as a separate aspect thereof" (p. 343). The BC-SC has two parts. The first part focuses on body cathexis (BC) and lists 46 body parts and functions. The second part is about self-cathexis (SC) and lists 55 items representing a sample of conceptual aspects of the self.

PSYCHOMETRIC PROPERTIES: The authors conducted extensive pre-liminary work with the BC-SC to eliminate unsatisfactory items. They administered the scale to college students. Split-half reliability tests for the BC and SC showed correlations ranging from 0.78 to 0.92. Subjects had a "moderate tendency to cathect their body to the same degree and in the same direction that they cathect their self" (Secord & Jourard, 1953, pp. 345-346). Balogun (1986) conducted a study to examine reliability of the BC-SC. He administered the scales to 50 female college students twice within a 2-week interval. The correlation between pre and post scores was 0.89 (p. 930). Several investigators have modified the BC-SC to fit their research interests. Some have been interested in the emotional impact of changes in oral health. Rudy, Guckes, Li, McCarthy, and Brahim (1993), who studied edentulism with older persons, adapted five items from a modification of the BC-SC to develop an orofacial cathexis scale.

PROCEDURE: Respondents are asked to consider each item listed and circle the number that "best represents your feelings according to the following scale: 1. Have strong feelings and wish change could somehow be made. 2. Don't like, but can put up with. 3. Have no particular feelings one way or the other. 4. Am satisfied. 5. Consider myself fortunate" (Secord & Jourard, 1953, p. 344).

SAMPLE BC ITEMS: "hair, waist, legs, sex activities" (Secord & Jourard, 1953, p. 344).

SAMPLE SC ITEMS: "last name, conscience, emotional control, ability to accept criticism" (Secord & Jourard, 1953, p. 344).

SCORING: The total BC score is obtained by summing the scores for the 46 items and dividing by 46. For total SC, sum the scores for the 55 items and divide by 55.

SOURCE: The items for the BC-SC and instructions for administration are printed in Secord and Jourard (1953).

REFERENCES

Balogun, J. A. (1986). Reliability and construct validity of the Body Cathexis Scale. *Perceptual and Motor Skills, 62,* 927-935.

Rudy, S. F., Guckes, A. D., Li, S., McCarthy, G. R., & Brahim, J. S. (1993). Body and orofacial cathexis in edentulous complete-denture-wearers. *Clinical Nursing Research, 2,* 296-308.

Secord, P., & Jourard, S. (1953). The appraisal of body cathexis and the self. *Journal of Consulting Psychology, 17,* 343-347.

BODY WORRIES AND BODY DISCOMFORTS TESTS (BW-BD)

AUTHORS: Robert Plutchik, M. Bakur Weiner, and Hope Conte
ADDRESS: Hope Conte, PhD
            Professor of Psychiatry
            Albert Einstein College of Medicine
            Department of Psychiatry
            Bronx Municipal Hospital Center
            Pelham Parkway South and Eastchester Road
            Bronx, NY 10461

DESCRIPTION: The Body Worries and Body Discomforts Tests (BW-BD) were designed as companion indexes of body image. The tests tap the frequencies of worries about and discomforts of the body. When they designed the measures, the authors reasoned that bodily concerns as reflected by discomforts and worries represented one aspect of body image (Plutchik, Bakur Weiner, & Conte, 1971, p. 345). The Body Worries form has 15 items that focus on concerns such as headache, palpitations, breathing, and indigestion. The Body Discomforts form asks the respondents to indicate which of 23 parts of their bodies are painful or give them discomfort.

PSYCHOMETRIC PROPERTIES: The authors tested the instruments with 165 individuals in six subgroups: senior center members, nursing home residents, former psychiatric patients, geriatric patients, psychiatric patients, and university students. The two tests were correlated for both male subjects ($n = 60$, 0.85) and female subjects ($n = 105$; 0.62). Split-half reliability estimates ranged from 0.86 to 0.95. Validity of the tests was supported to some extent by the differences between scores associated with known groups. For example, females had more discomforts and worries than males, and members of the group with the highest scores for worries and discomforts were female and diagnosed as schizophrenic (Plutchik et al., 1971, p. 349).

PROCEDURE: The tests may be administered verbally or as paper-and-pencil instruments.

SAMPLE ITEMS: "Do you worry about getting bad headaches?" and "Do you worry that your heart will race or thump for no reason?" (Plutchik et al., 1971, p. 345).

SCORING: Responses to items on both instruments are *never* (0), *sometimes* (1), or *often* (2). A higher score reflects more disturbed body image.

SOURCE: A copy of the Body Worries form appears in Plutchik et al. (1971). The list of parts for the Body Discomfort instrument also appears in Plutchik et al. (1971, p. 345).

REFERENCE

Plutchik, R., Bakur Weiner, M., & Conte, H. (1971). Studies of body image. I. Body worries and body discomfort. *Journal of Gerontology, 26,* 344-350.

BORG SCALE OR RATING OF PERCEIVED EXERTION (RPE)

AUTHORS: Gunnar A. V. Borg and Bruce J. Noble
ADDRESSES: Gunnar A. V. Borg
            Department of Psychology
            Box 5602
            S-114 86 Stockholm, Sweden

            Bruce J. Noble
            Department of Physical and Health Education
            University of Wyoming
            Laramie, WY 82071

DESCRIPTION: The Rating of Perceived Exertion (RPE) is a scale used when an investigator or clinician wants to obtain a simple, direct estimate of subjective physical strain. Borg (1982) said that the RPE "integrates various information, including many signals elicited from the peripheral working muscles and joints, from the central cardiovascular and respiratory functions, and from the central nervous system" (p. 377). Ratings on the scale range from 6 to 20. There are seven "adjectival-adverbial anchor expressions," corresponding to odd numbers on the scale and ranging from *very, very light* to *very, very hard* (p. 378). During the development of the scale, the numbers and terms were manipulated so that the RPE had a "linear relationship with heart rate" for most subjects. The RPE was constructed, using young and middle-aged samples, so that heart rate would be about 10 times the RPE (Borg & Noble, 1974, p. 139). The scale has also been used with older men (Blumenthal et al., 1991) and women (Hassemen, Ceci, & Backman, 1992), however, and has been found effective as a "moderator of exercise intensity" (Hassemen et al., 1992, p. 464). Compared with younger persons, elders rate their exertion higher in relation to their heart rates (Borg & Noble, 1974, p. 144). Therefore, when using the scale with frail elders, RPE standards would be conservatively modified. Borg scales have also been used to measure pain (Law, McIntosh, Morrison, & Baptiste, 1987) and dyspnea (Killian, Summers, Jones, & Campbell, 1992; Lush, Janson-Bjerklie, Carrieri, & Lovejoy, 1988).

PSYCHOMETRIC PROPERTIES: In many studies, investigators have found correlations between RPE ratings and heart rates (Borg, 1982, p. 378).

Validity has also been supported by the correspondence between RPE ratings and measurements of physical work capacity (Borg & Noble, 1974, p. 140). Ratings on the scale, in relation to workload, have been higher in "groups of patients" than in "normal reference groups" (Borg & Noble, 1974, p. 141). Borg and Noble (1974) have shown test-retest reliability at 2 to 4 weeks, ranging between 0.88 and 0.98 (p. 140). Environmental heat and medications have effects on RPEs (p. 143), and effects from psychological variables have also been observed (Boutcher, Fleischer-Cutian, & Gines, 1988).

PROCEDURE: Applications for the RPE are varied. One might use the scale to monitor exertion during a walking program for elders. Following medical clearance and consent, one would instruct the subject about the RPE, saying something like the following:

> When we are walking, we want to be sure you are comfortable. We have this chart that will help us (show RPE scale). Along this line there are numbers from 6 to 20 and next to the numbers, words that describe how *light* or *hard* the walking is. We do not want it to be hard for you (point to #15). Neither do we want it to be very very light (point to #7). We would like your effort to be between fairly light (point to #9) and somewhat hard (point to #13). While we are walking, from time to time, I am going to ask you how you are doing, and you will give me a number.

SAMPLE ITEMS: 9 is *very light,* 11 is *fairly light,* and 13 is *somewhat hard* (Borg & Noble, 1974, p. 138).

SCORING: The RPE is treated statistically as an ordinal scale (Borg & Noble, 1974). Borg (1982) has also constructed a scale with ratio properties (p. 30).

SOURCE: The scale is popular internationally. It has been translated into French, German, Japanese, Hebrew, and Russian (Borg, 1982, p. 378). It is reprinted in Borg (1982) and Borg and Noble (1974).

REFERENCES

Blumenthal, J. A., Emery, C. F., Madden, D. J., Schniebolk, S., Riddle, M. W., Cobb, F. R., Higginbotham, M., & Coleman, R. E. (1991). Effects of exercise training on bone density in older men and women. *Journal of the American Geriatrics Society, 39,* 1065-1070.

Borg, G. A. V. (1982). Psychophysiological bases of perceived exertion. *Medicine and Science in Sports and Exercise, 14,* 377-381.

Borg, G. A. V., & Noble, B. J. (1974). Perceived exertion. In J. P. Wilmore (Ed.), *Exercise and Sports Sciences Reviews* (Vol. 2, pp. 131-153). New York: Academic Press.

Boutcher, S. H., Fleischer-Cutian, L. A., & Gines, S. D. (1988). The effects of self-presentation on perceived exertion. *Journal of Sport and Exercise Physiology, 10*, 270-280.

Hassemen, P., Ceci, R., & Backman, L. (1992). Exercise training for older women: A training method and its influences on physical and cognitive performance. *European Journal of Applied Physiology, 64*, 460-466.

Killian, K. J., Summers, E., Jones, N. L., & Campbell, E. J. M. (1992). Dyspnea and leg effort during incremental cycle ergometry. *American Review of Respiratory Disease, 145*, 1339-1345.

Law, M., McIntosh, J., Morrison, L., & Baptiste, S. (1987). A comparison of two pain measurement scales: Their clinical value. *Canadian Journal of Rehabilitation, 1*(1), 55-58.

Lush, M. T., Janson-Bjerklie, S., Carrieri, V. K., & Lovejoy, N. (1988). Dyspnea in the ventilator-assisted patient. *Heart and Lung, 17*, 528-535.

BRADEN SCALE FOR PREDICTING PRESSURE SORE RISK

AUTHORS: Barbara J. Braden and Nancy Bergstrom

ADDRESS: Barbara J. Braden, PhD, RN, and
            Nancy Bergstrom, PhD, RN
            College of Nursing
            University of Nebraska Medical Center
            600 South 42 Street
            Omaha, NE 68198-5330

DESCRIPTION: The Braden Scale for Predicting Pressure Sore Risk was designed for early identification of persons at risk for pressure sore development. It has six one-item subscales used to assess variables associated with risk for impaired skin integrity. Respondents evaluate (a) sensory perception (the ability to respond to discomfort), (b) moisture (degree of skin exposure to moisture), (c) activity (degree of physical activity), (d) mobility (ability independently to change body position), (e) nutrition (usual food intake pattern), and (f) friction (the extent to which the person's skin is exposed to shearing forces).

PSYCHOMETRIC PROPERTIES: Interrater reliability for the scale was tested with registered nurse (RN), licensed practical nurse (LPN), and nurse's aide (NA) raters. Percentages of agreement ranged from a low of 11% for NA raters to a high of 88% for RN raters. Correlations for pairs of scores reached 0.99 for RNs, 0.94 for LPNs, and 0.83 for NAs (Bergstrom, Braden, Laguzza, & Holman, 1987, p. 207). Bergstrom and Braden (1992) conducted a prospective study of 200 individuals newly admitted to nursing homes and at risk for pressure sores. Predictors of pressure sore development included score on the scale, diastolic blood pressure, temperature, dietary protein intake, and age. "The Braden Scale score reported the week prior to the first pressure sore was the strongest predictor of pressure sore development" (Bergstrom & Braden, 1992, p. 756). The tool has been tested in intensive care units, medical-surgical units, patients' homes, and long-term care. Thus, it can be useful to track progress across settings.

PROCEDURE: The scale is presented in a 5 × 6 table on one page, including space for subscale scores and total score. The observer conducts a direct assessment and also consults the subject's health record. The observer matches the scale's descriptive phrases with observations of the subject's circumstances.

SAMPLE ITEM:

Moisture: degree to which skin is exposed to moisture.

---

1   *Constantly Moist:* Skin is kept moist almost constantly by perspiration, urine, etc. Dampness is detected every time patient is moved or turned.

2   *Very Moist:* Skin is often but not always moist. Linen must be changed at least once a shift.

3   *Occasionally Moist:* Skin is occasionally moist, requiring an extra linen change approximately once a day.

4   *Rarely Moist:* Skin is usually dry, linen only requires changing at routine intervals.

(Braden & Bergstrom, 1988)

SCORING: Scores range from 6 to 23. Higher scores indicate less risk. The observer rates the subscales from 1 (*most risk*) to 4 (*least risk*). The highest score for the friction/shear scale is 3. On the basis of data from their study published in 1992, Bergstrom and Braden concluded that "elderly nursing home residents with scores on the Braden Scale below 12 are at high risk for pressure sore development. . . . Scores between 13 and 15 reflect moderate risk. . . . Scores greater than 16 or 17 probably represent mild risk" (p. 756).

SOURCE: Professors Braden and Bergstrom hold the copyright for the Braden Scale. Prospective users should contact them for a copy and for permission to use the scale.

REFERENCES

Bergstrom, N., & Braden, B. (1992). A prospective study of pressure sore risk among institutionalized elderly. *Journal of the American Geriatrics Society, 40,* 747-758.

Bergstrom, N., Braden, B., Laguzza, A., & Holman, V. (1987). The Braden Scale for Predicting Pressure Sore Risk. *Nursing Research, 36,* 205-210.

Braden, B., & Bergstrom, N. (1988). *The Braden Scale for Predicting Pressure Sore Risk.* (Available from the authors at address listed above)

BRIEF AGITATION RATING SCALE (BARS)

AUTHORS: Sanford I. Finkel, John S. Lyons, and Rachel L. Anderson
ADDRESS: Sanford I. Finkel, MD
             Northwestern University Medical School
             Department of Psychiatry and Behavioral Sciences
             303 East Ohio Street, Suite 550
             Chicago, IL 60611-3317

DESCRIPTION: The Brief Agitation Rating Scale (BARS) was developed to "quickly and effectively assess behavioral problems in order to design and evaluate treatment and management plans" for elderly patients (Finkel, Lyons, & Anderson, 1993a, p. 51). It is a 10-item scale derived from the longer Cohen-Mansfield Agitation Inventory (CMAI; see entry in this book).

PSYCHOMETRIC PROPERTIES: The authors of BARS used the Cohen-Mansfield conceptual framework for their tool, including the three dimensions of physically aggressive, physically nonaggressive, and verbally agitated behaviors. In one long-term care facility, registered nurses and certified nurse assistants using the CMAI rated 232 (196 females) residents for whom they had been the "main caregiver." The average age of the sample was 86, with age range from 65 to 102 years. Ratings for 20 randomly selected residents were tested for interrater agreement. Items selected for the BARS reflected the three dimensions tapped by the CMAI and were those items that had high item-total correlations and high interrater reliability. Correlations between scores for BARS items and scores on the full CMAI were similar on three work shifts (0.95, 0.94, 0.95). The intraclass correlation for agreement between raters for the 10-item BARS was 0.73, higher than for the full 29-item CMAI (0.41; Finkel et al., 1993a, p. 51). Alpha coefficients for the BARS (range 0.74 to 0.82) were lower than for the CMAI (0.86 to 0.91). To assess validity for the BARS, scores were correlated with scores on two other behavior scales for 40 residents across three shifts. Same-shift correlations were significant at the 0.05 level or better ($r = 0.33$ to 0.53) for days and evenings. Correlations between ratings made on different shifts and between two ratings made on the night shift were low. The authors suggested further validation studies (Finkel et al., 1993a, p. 52).

PROCEDURE: "Ratings should be accomplished by a caregiver who has had the opportunity to observe the resident in question over a two week period of time" (Finkel, Lyons, & Anderson, 1993b, p. 2).

SAMPLE ITEMS: "Hitting," "Repetitious sentences or questions," and "Pacing/aimless wandering" (Finkel et al., 1993b, p. 5).

SCORING: Each behavior is rated by frequency of occurrence, using the following scale: 1 = *none,* 2 = *once in 2 weeks,* 3 = *2 or 3 times in 2 weeks,* 4 = *once a week,* 5 = *2 to 3 times a week,* 6 = *once a day,* and 7 = *several times a day* (Finkel et al., 1993b, p. 2). Range for a total BARS score is 10 to 70. Several different ways of deriving scores from the ratings are suggested in the manual.

SOURCE: The manual and scale are available from the authors. Permission to reprint the scale must be obtained from the *Journal of the American Geriatrics Society.*

REFERENCES

Finkel, S. I., Lyons, J. S., & Anderson, R. L. (1993a). A Brief Agitation Rating Scale (BARS) for nursing home elderly. *Journal of the American Geriatrics Society, 41,* 50-52.

Finkel, S. I., Lyons, J. S., & Anderson, R. L. (1993b). *The Brief Agitation Rating Scale (BARS) manual.* (Available from the authors at address listed above)

BRIEF COGNITIVE RATING SCALE (BCRS)

AUTHORS: Barry Reisberg and Steven H. Ferris
ADDRESS: Barry Reisberg, MD, Clinical Director
            Aging and Dementia Research Center
            New York University Medical Center
            550 Fifth Avenue
            New York, NY 10016

DESCRIPTION: The Brief Cognitive Rating Scale—Axis I-IV (BCRS) is an instrument designed to assess the extent of cognitive impairment in four clinical areas (termed *axes*) using specific criteria (Reisberg & Ferris, 1988, p. 629). A clinician using the scale rates concentration, recent memory, past memory, and orientation, using a standardized approach. Originally, a fifth axis of the BCRS was used to assess functioning and self-care. That axis became a 16-stage ordinal scale for measuring functional change known as the Functional Assessment Staging (FAST). Ratings on this BCRS, which is part of a staging system for clinical assessment of aging and of Alzheimer's disease (AD), correspond to stages of the Global Deterioration Scale (see entry in this book). The BCRS has been used widely in investigations of the efficacy of pharmacological agents in the treatment of cognitive impairment associated with AD (p. 629).

PSYCHOMETRIC PROPERTIES: Correlations between scores for 40 assessments made simultaneously, but rated independently, demonstrated inter-rater reliability (range 0.82 to 0.97; Reisberg, Sclan, Franssen, Kluger, & Ferris, 1994, p. S194). In two studies of nursing home residents ($N = 408$), 93% of ratings made independently by charge nurses ($N = 31$) were in exact agreement or within 1 point of exact agreement; correlations between ratings made by nurses and social workers ranged between 0.76 and 0.82 (Cohen-Mansfield, Marx, & Rosenthal, 1990). Correlations for baseline and follow-up scores were 0.96 for the total BCRS and ranged from 0.82 to 0.86 for the test-retest reliability of the four axes' scores (Reisberg & Ferris, 1988, p. 631).

PROCEDURE: Data for the BCRS are gathered in a "semi-structured" clinical interview "conducted in the presence of the spouse or primary caregiver, whenever possible" (Reisberg & Ferris, 1988, p. 629). Questions to introduce each assessment area are suggested in the scoring guidelines (pp. 633-636). For example, the task to elicit data about concentration is introduced with questions such as "How far did you go in school?" and "How are you at subtraction?" Depending on the level of decline, the subject is asked to recite the months backwards, perform serial subtractions, or count backward, or forward, by 2s or 1s.

SAMPLE ITEM:

Axis I: Concentration.

---

1 = No objective or subjective evidence of deficit in concentration.

2 = Subjective decrement in concentration ability.

3 = Minor objective signs of poor concentration (e.g., on subtraction of serial 7s from 100).

4 = Definite concentration deficit for persons of their background (e.g., marked deficit on serial 7s; frequent deficit in subtraction of serial 4s from 40).

5 = Marked concentration deficit (e.g., giving months backwards or serial 2s from 20).

6 = Forgets the concentration task. Frequently begins to count forward when asked to count backward from 10 by 1s.

7 = Marked difficulty counting to 10 by 1s.

(Reisberg & Ferris, 1988, p. 632)

SCORING: For each axis, the rater circles the highest score achieved by the subject.

SOURCE: The BCRS is reprinted in Reisberg and Ferris (1988) and Reisberg et al. (1994).

REFERENCES

Cohen-Mansfield, J., Marx, M. S., & Rosenthal, A. S. (1990). Dementia and agitation in nursing home residents: How are they related? *Psychology and Aging, 5,* 3-8.

Reisberg, B., & Ferris, S. H. (1988). *Psychopharmacological Bulletin, 24,* 629-636.

Reisberg, B., Sclan, S. G., Franssen, E., Kluger, A., & Ferris, S. (1994). Dementia staging in chronic care populations. *Alzheimer Disease and Associated Disorders, 8*(Suppl. 1), S188-S205.

BURDEN INTERVIEW (BURDEN)

AUTHORS: Steven H. Zarit and Judy M. Zarit
ADDRESS: Gerontology Center
            College of Health and Human Development
            The Pennsylvania State University
            240 Henderson Building South
            University Park, PA 16802

DESCRIPTION: The Burden Interview is a 22-item scale designed to assess the extent to which caregivers of elderly and disabled persons perceive their roles and responsibilities as having adverse effects on their "health, personal and social life, finances, and emotional well-being" (Whitlatch, Zarit, & von Eye, 1991, p. 10). It is intended for use when the clinician or researcher wants "a single summary measure of caregivers' appraisals of the impact their involvement has had on their lives" (Zarit & Zarit, 1990, p. 8). The authors believed that the Burden Interview should not be the sole measure of the "caregiver's emotional state," however. They suggested that "clinical observations and other instruments such as measures of depression should be used to supplement the measure" (p. 8). Two subscales have been derived from the Burden Interview: the Personal Strain subscale and the Role Strain subscale (Whitlatch et al., 1991, p. 14). One of the 22 items measures overall burden.

PSYCHOMETRIC PROPERTIES: Estimates of reliability for the Burden Interview have been reported for a doctoral dissertation and in a paper presented at a meeting of the Gerontological Society of America (alpha coefficients = 0.88 and 0.91; test-retest reliability = 0.71; cited in Zarit & Zarit, 1990, p. 8). Anthony-Bergstone, Zarit, and Gatz (1988) estimated validity with correlations between Burden Interview scores and global ratings of burden (0.71) and scores on the Brief Symptom Inventory (Derogatis, Lipman, Covl, Richels, & Uhlenhuth, 1970; 0.41).

PROCEDURE: The observer interviews the caregiver, who reports the frequency of the feelings he or she has experienced.

SAMPLE ITEMS: "Do you feel that your social life has suffered because you are caring for your relative?" and "Do you feel that you have lost control of your life since your relative's illness?" (Zarit & Zarit, 1990, p. 10).

SCORING: The possible responses to 21 of the items are 0 (*never*), 1 (*rarely*), 2 (*sometimes*), 3 (*quite frequently*), and 4 (*nearly always*). For overall burden, the response may be 0 (*not at all*), 1 (*a little*), 2 (*moderately*), 3 (*quite a bit*), or 4 (*extremely*). The sum of the item scores is the total Burden Interview score.

SOURCE: The instrument and instructions for its use are available for a small fee from the Gerontology Center at Pennsylvania State University at the above address.

REFERENCES

Anthony-Bergstone, C., Zarit, S. H., & Gatz, M. (1988). Symptoms of psychological distress among caregivers of dementia patients. *Psychology and Aging, 3,* 245-248.

Derogatis, L. R., Lipman, R. S., Covl, L., Richels, K., & Uhlenhuth, E. R. (1970). Dimensions of outpatient neurotic pathology: Comparison of a clinical versus an empirical assessment. *Journal of Consulting and Clinical Psychology, 34,* 164-171.

Whitlatch, C. J., Zarit, S. H., & von Eye, A. (1991). Efficacy of interventions with caregivers: A reanalysis. *Gerontologist, 31,* 9-14.

Zarit, S. H., & Zarit, J. M. (1990). *The Memory and Behavior Checklist and the Burden Interview.* (Available from the authors at address listed above)

CAGE QUESTIONNAIRE

AUTHORS: J. A. Ewing and B. A. Rouse, with further development by Demmie Mayfield, Gail McLeod, and Patricia Hall

ADDRESS: Demmie G. Mayfield, MD
Audie L. Murphy Veterans Hospital
7400 Merton Minter Boulevard
San Antonio, TX 78284

DESCRIPTION: The CAGE Questionnaire is an alcoholism screening test. Compared with other screening methods available for alcoholism, it is easy to administer. The tool's four items are relatively nonthreatening. Its title is an acronym for key words in the questions. The CAGE has been used widely by nurses and other health care providers.

PSYCHOMETRIC PROPERTIES: Building on the work of Ewing and Rouse (1970), Mayfield, McLeod, and Hall (1974) conducted studies to evaluate the tool's "usefulness" with 366 psychiatric patients admitted to a psychiatric service of a VA hospital over a 1-year period. Categorical ratings (alcoholic or nonalcoholic) based on multidisciplinary diagnostic evaluations were made post discharge by a social worker. These ratings were correlated with the patient's response to each of the CAGE items. Thirty-nine percent of the patients were categorized as alcoholics and 61% as nonalcoholics. When all four items of the tool were used as criteria for positive screening, there were no false positives, but only 37 out of approximately 142 alcoholics were categorized as alcoholic (phi = 0.65). When only two or three responses were used as criteria, the correlation coefficients were higher (phi = .89). Many alcoholics did not answer "yes" to the item "Have people *annoyed* you by criticizing your drinking?" Consequently, the item had "substantially lower power as a predictive criterion" (Mayfield et al., 1974, p. 1122).

PROCEDURE: To *screen* for alcoholism, the respondent is asked to provide a "yes" or "no" response to each item.

CAGE ITEMS:

1. Have you ever felt you should *cut down* on your drinking?
2. Have people *annoyed* you by criticizing your drinking?
3. Have you ever felt bad or *guilty* about your drinking?
4. Have you ever had a drink first thing in the morning to steady your nerves or get rid of a hang-over (*eye-opener*)? (Mayfield et al., 1974, p. 1121)

SCORING: The evaluation of the instrument showed that it was not as sensitive when a four-item criterion was used as it was when a two- or three-item cutoff for screening positive was adopted.

SOURCE: The questionnaire is in the public domain.

REFERENCES

Ewing, J. A., & Rouse, B. A. (1970, February). *Identifying the hidden alcoholic.* Paper presented at the 29th International Congress on Alcoholism and Drug Dependence, Sydney, Australia.

Mayfield, D., McLeod, G., & Hall, P. (1974). The CAGE questionnaire: Validation of a new alcoholism screening instrument. *American Journal of Psychiatry, 131,* 1121-1123.

CANTRIL'S LADDER OR LADDER SCALE

AUTHORS: F. P. Kilpatrick and Hadley Cantril

DESCRIPTION: The Self-Anchoring Ladder Scale is a "self-defined continuum anchored at either end in terms of personal perception" (Kilpatrick & Cantril, 1960, p. 160). The self-anchoring method, which is a general approach to measurement, is derived from the notion that "each of us lives and operates in the world and through the self, both *as perceived*" (Kilpatrick & Cantril, 1960, p. 158). The key point here is that "unique perceptions, goals and values of each individual are taken into account" (p. 159). The scale is readily understandable.

PSYCHOMETRIC PROPERTIES: Kilpatrick and Cantril (1960) reported that a 10-interval scale provided "a satisfactory degree of discrimination" (p. 160).

PROCEDURE: Before administration, a respondent is asked to describe what would be the very best or ideal way of life and, after that is clearly determined, to describe what would be the very worst way of life for him or her. Descriptions are recorded as accurately as possible. The scale is then presented as a picture of a ladder with 11 rungs numbered 0 through 10. The respondent is advised that 10 is the best way of life and 0 the worst way of life as he or she has just described it. The respondent is then asked, "Where on this ladder would you say you are now?" The step number response is the "location of the self in the now" (Kilpatrick & Cantril, 1960, p. 159). From this reference point, other scaling and interviewing may proceed, depending on the purpose of the assessment, intervention, or research.

SAMPLE ITEMS: Other perspectives can be substituted for "way of life" in the administration of the ladder: for example, best and worst possible futures (i.e., hopes/aspirations and fears/worries about health, values, relatives, family, and the future of the country). A respondent can also be asked to choose a step number representing perception of "self" at a time in the past as well as a time in the future.

SCORING: The numbers on the scale represent a continuum, with the top and bottom self-defined. The method can be used both with individuals and with large samples. The responses chosen may be treated statistically as ordinal numbers.

SOURCE: This scale and others like it are reprinted in Kilpatrick and Cantril (1960).

REFERENCE

Kilpatrick, F. P., & Cantril, H. (1960). Self-anchoring scaling: A measure of individuals' unique reality worlds. *Journal of Individual Psychology, 16,* 158-173.

CAREGIVER REACTION ASSESSMENT (CRA)

AUTHORS: Charles W. Given, Barbara Given, Manfred Stommel,
            Clare Collins, Sharon King, and Susan Franklin
ADDRESS: Charles W. Given, PhD
            Michigan State University
            Department of Family Practice
            B-109 Clinical Center
            East Lansing, MI 48823-1313

DESCRIPTION: The Caregiver Reaction Assessment (CRA) is a multi-dimensional 24-item instrument constructed to "assess the reactions of family members caring for elderly persons with physical impairments, Alzheimer's Disease (AD) and cancer" (Given et al., 1992, p. 271). The instrument has five distinct subscales: esteem, family support, finance, schedule, and health.

PSYCHOMETRIC PROPERTIES: The team of authors used clinical interviews and the literature to identify items that reflected reactions to caregiving. The tool was tested with exploratory factor analysis of data gathered from a sample of 377 caregivers of persons with physical impairments and AD. Alpha coefficients for subscales ranged between 0.80 and 0.90. To confirm equivalency of the measure across diseases (AD vs. cancer) and relationships (spouse vs. nonspouse), as well as longitudinally (caregivers of physically disabled), the authors used confirmatory factor analysis to demonstrate a stable subscale structure (Stommel, Wang, Given, & Given, 1992). Construct validity was also supported by subscale correlations ($N = 754$) with patient dependency in ADLs and caregiver depression (Given et al., 1992, pp. 281-282).

PROCEDURE: Respondents are instructed to circle one of five responses for each item: *strongly agree, agree, neither agree or disagree, disagree,* or *strongly disagree.*

SAMPLE ITEMS: "I have to stop in the middle of my work" and "Caring for _____ is important to me" (Stommel et al., 1992, p. 403).

SCORING: Items are coded 1 = *strongly disagree* to 5 = *strongly agree.* Five items are scored in reverse.

SOURCE: Copies of the instrument and permission for its use are available from the authors.

REFERENCES

Given, C. W., Given, B., Stommel, M., Collins, C., King, S., & Franklin, S. (1992). The Caregiver Reaction Assessment (CRA) for caregivers to persons with chronic physical and mental impairments. *Research in Nursing and Health, 15,* 271-283.

Stommel, M., Wang, S., Given, C. W., & Given, B. (1992). Confirmatory factor analysis (CFA) as a method to assess measurement equivalence. *Research in Nursing and Health, 15,* 399-405.

CHRONIC RESPIRATORY DISEASE QUESTIONNAIRE (CRQ)

AUTHORS: Gordon H. Guyatt, Leslie B. Berman, Marie Townsend, Stewart O. Pugsley, and Larry W. Chambers

ADDRESS: Dr. Gordon H. Guyatt
Clinical Epidemiology and Biostatistics
McMaster University Health Sciences Centre
1200 Main Street West
Hamilton, Ontario L8N 3Z5, Canada

DESCRIPTION: The Chronic Respiratory Disease Questionnaire (CRQ) was designed to measure the quality of life of persons with chronic respiratory problems (Guyatt, Berman, Townsend, Pugsley, & Chambers, 1987, p. 773).

Like its counterpart, the Chronic Heart Failure Index Questionnaire (CHQ; Guyatt, Bombardier, & Tugwell, 1986; see "Source" section below), it was intended for use in clinical trials. The beginning of this 20-item questionnaire focuses on dyspnea. With specific prompting from the interviewer, the respondent identifies five day-to-day activities that he or she associates with shortness of breath and then ranks them for importance. For each of the five activities chosen, the respondent rates the extent of dyspnea experienced in the last 2 weeks. The other items have 7-point scale responses and focus on fatigue (four items), emotional function (seven items), and mastery (four items). *Mastery* is defined by the authors as "the patient's feeling of control over the disease" (Guyatt et al., 1987, p. 773).

PSYCHOMETRIC PROPERTIES: Items generated by experts and derived from the literature were evaluated by 100 randomly selected patients with chronic airflow limitation. They were asked "to identify items that were problems for them, and to rate the importance of each problem" (Guyatt et al., 1987, p. 774). The investigators multiplied frequency by importance, and items with the highest results were chosen for the fatigue, emotional function, and mastery components of the instrument. For the dyspnea component, items were developed so that responses could be specific to individual patients. The CRQ was administered six times at 2-week intervals to 25 patients with "stable" chronic airflow limitations. Test-retest reliability was supported by similar mean scores for all four dimensions at each administration (p. 774). To demonstrate responsiveness of the CRQ, the authors administered it to get baseline scores and subsequently to get follow-up scores for two small samples of patients ($ns = 13$ and 28) who were expected to show post-treatment improvement. With "only small improvements in spirometric values," CRQ scores in all four dimensions were "substantially better at follow-up" (p. 774). Responsiveness was further demonstrated by comparisons of pre- and post-treatment CRQ scores with scores on similar measures (p. 775).

PROCEDURE: The questionnaire is administered in a clinical interview. CRQ forms are detailed and require some advanced preparation by the interviewer. The authors have prepared "Background Information and Interviewing Tips" (see "Source" section below) for this purpose. The interviewer has a complete text to follow on the CRQ interview form. To facilitate responses, the interviewer provides the subject with specific color-coded cards on which the seven possible responses appear in large print. Initial administration of the CRQ takes about 30 minutes. Follow-up administration takes a little less time (Guyatt et al., 1987, p. 774). The day-to-day activities identified by the respondent at baseline are used again for the first five items of the follow-up questionnaire. The authors suggested that the respondent be informed of his or her baseline responses before answering each of the items in the follow-up interview (Guyatt, Berman, Townsend, & Taylor, 1985).

SAMPLE ITEM:

How often during the past 2 weeks did you have a feeling of fear or panic when you had difficulty getting your breath?

1. All of the time
2. Most of the time
3. A good bit of the time
4. Some of the time
5. A little of the time
6. Hardly any of the time
7. None of the time (Guyatt et al., 1987, p. 777)

SCORING: Scores for each of the four dimensions are "standardized on a ten-point scale" (Guyatt et al., 1987, p. 774). For example, the total possible subscore for dyspnea is 35. To calculate the score for that dimension, one would divide the sum of the five obtained scores for dyspnea by 3.5. The scoring guidelines provided by the authors include scores recommended for judging "clinically important differences" and a formula for scoring missing data.

SOURCE: The CRQ is reprinted in Guyatt et al. (1987). However, the user needs both baseline and follow-up interview forms, CRQ response sheets, response cards, and the mimeographed "Background Information and Interviewing Tips," which includes guidelines for scoring. An audiotape to train interviewers is also recommended. These materials are available from the author for a fee.

To administer the Chronic Heart Failure Index Questionnaire (CHQ; Guyatt et al., 1986), an instrument that is the same as the CRQ except for one item, the clinician or investigator needs a CHQ packet.

REFERENCES

Guyatt, G. H., Berman, L. B., Townsend, M., Pugsley, S. O., & Chambers, L. W. (1987). A measure of quality of life for clinical trials in chronic lung disease. *Thorax, 42,* 773-778.

Guyatt, G. H., Berman, L. B., Townsend, M., & Taylor, D. W. (1985). Should subjects see their previous responses? *Journal of Chronic Diseases, 38,* 1003-1007.
Guyatt, G. H., Bombardier, C., & Tugwell, P. X. (1986). Measuring disease-specific quality of life in clinical trials. *Canadian Medical Association Journal, 134,* 889-895.

CLIFTON ASSESSMENT PROCEDURES FOR THE ELDERLY (CAPE), COGNITIVE ASSESSMENT SCALE (CAS), AND BEHAVIOR RATING SCALE (BRS)

AUTHORS: Anne H. Pattie and Christopher J. Gilleard
ADDRESS: Christopher J. Gilleard
            Department of Psychology
            Springfield University Hospital
            61 Glenburnie Road
            Tooting SW17 7DJ, London, United Kingdom

DESCRIPTION: The Clifton Assessment Procedures for the Elderly (CAPE) has been used to predict clinical outcomes, select candidates for rehabilitation, and categorize individuals in terms of their dependency needs. The CAPE has two independent scales that may be used together or separately: the Cognitive Assessment Scale (CAS) and the Behavior Rating Scale (BRS). The CAS is a brief psychological test for evaluating "the existence and degree of impairment in mental functioning" (Pattie & Gilleard, 1979, p. 1). It is made up of three components: information-orientation (12 items), mental abilities (4 items), and a timed psychomotor paper-and-pencil test. The BRS provides "an overall measurement of an individual's behavioural disability level" (p. 1). It was derived from the Stockton Geriatric Rating Scale (Meer & Baker, 1966) and initially published by the authors in 1977 as the Shortened Stockton Geriatric Rating Scale (Gilleard & Pattie, 1977). The BRS is an 18-item instrument designed to be completed by caregiving staff members or relatives. The items assess physical disability, apathy, communication difficulty, and socially disturbing behavior (Gilleard, 1994, p. 55).

PSYCHOMETRIC PROPERTIES: There is an extensive discussion of the psychometric properties of both the CAS and BRS in the CAPE manual (Pattie & Gilleard, 1979). Short-term stability of the CAS subtests was demonstrated with a sample ($N = 38$) of acutely ill elders tested on admission and retested several days later ($r = 0.79$ to 0.87). Correlations of test-retest scores on CAS subtests for long-stay psychogeriatric patients ranged from 0.56 to 0.90 (Pattie & Gilleard, 1979, p. 21). Scores for "non-pathological elderly groups" were also relatively stable ($r = 0.69$ to 0.84). Correlations of scores assigned by independent raters for the four components of the BRS ranged from 0.70 to 0.91 for physical disability, 0.81 to 0.87 for apathy, 0.45 to 0.72 for communication difficulties, and 0.69 to 0.88 for social disturbance (Pattie & Gilleard, 1979, p. 22). Validity of the CAS was supported through comparisons between CAS scores and scores on the Wechsler Adult Intelligence Test Memory scale (Savage, Britton, Bolton, & Hall, 1973; Pattie & Gilleard, 1979, p. 23) and by analysis of the CAS scores of known groups. Validity of the BRS is supported by scores for known groups that required different levels of support and service (pp. 26-27). Factor structure for the BRS has differed depending on the sample tested. Predictive validity for the CAS was demonstrated with classification of psychiatric patients as either functional or organic and "discrimination between those discharged and those not" (Pattie & Gilleard, 1979, p. 14). BRS scores identified persons on "long-stay" wards who were candidates for rehabilitation. The grading system for CAPE was normed in studies of diverse samples ranging from community-dwelling well elders to institutionalized geriatric patients.

PROCEDURE: The observer needs to be thoroughly familiar with the CAS before proceeding. Performance is timed with a stopwatch or device with a second hand. A detailed script for administering the CAS and scoring criteria for each of the items are provided in the CAPE manual (Pattie & Gilleard, 1979). The BRS is completed by a caregiver. Responses refer to what the subject actually has done for the past several weeks, rather than what he or she might do.

SAMPLE CAS ITEM: "Will you write your name here for me?" (Pattie & Gilleard, 1979, p. 5).

SAMPLE BRS ITEM: "He/she is objectionable to others during the day (loud or constant talking, pilfering, soiling furniture, interfering with affairs of others) rarely or never (0), sometimes (1), frequently (2)" (Pattie & Gilleard, 1979, p. 9).

SCORING: There are scoring criteria for each item of the CAS in the manual (Pattie & Gilleard, 1979). The total BRS score is the sum of the subscores for physical disability (dependency), apathy, communication difficulty, and socially disturbing behavior. Data for both scales are recorded on the CAPE Report Form (Pattie & Gilleard, 1979) for summary purposes. Scores may be graded from A to E, representing varying levels of impairment and dependency: Grade A = no impairment and independence, Grade B = mild impairment with low dependency, Grade C = moderate impairment with medium dependency, Grade D = marked impairment and high dependency, and Grade E = severe impairment with maximum dependency. Grades C, D, and E have subcategories that further refine degrees of dependency (Pattie & Gilleard, 1979, pp. 10-12).

SOURCE: The instruments are copyrighted by the authors. The manual (Pattie & Gilleard, 1979) includes instructions, the instruments, and recording forms.

REFERENCES

Gilleard, C. (1994). Cognition and behavior. In I. Philp (Ed.), *Assessing elderly people in hospital and community* (pp. 51-58). London: Farrand.

Gilleard, C. J., & Pattie, A. H. (1977). The Stockton Geriatric Rating Scale: A shortened version with British normative data. *British Journal of Psychiatry, 131,* 90-94.

Meer, B., & Baker, J. A. (1966). The Stockton Geriatric Rating Scale. *Journal of Gerontology, 21,* 392-403.

Pattie, A. H., & Gilleard, C. J. (1979). *Manual of the Clifton Assessment Procedures for the Elderly (CAPE).* (Available from Hodder and Stoughton Educational, 338 Euston Road, London NW1 3BH, UK)

Savage, R. D., Britton, P. G., Bolton, N., & Hall, E. H. (1973). *Intellectual functioning in the aged.* London: Methuen.

CLINICAL DEMENTIA RATING (CDR)

AUTHORS: Charles P. Hughes, Leonard Berg, Warren L. Danziger, Lawrence A. Coben, and Ronald L. Martin

ADDRESS: Leonard Berg, MD
Professor of Neurology and Director
Washington University
Alzheimer's Disease Research Center
4488 Forest Park Boulevard
St. Louis, MO 63108-2293

DESCRIPTION: The Clinical Dementia Rating (CDR), an instrument developed at Washington University, was designed to rate cognitive impairment in each of six categories: (a) memory, (b) orientation, (c) judgment and problem solving, (d) community affairs, (e) home and hobbies, and (f) personal care. The CDR can be used "for comparing degrees of dementia from patient to patient and from institution to institution" (Berg, 1988, p. 637). It has been used "in longitudinal studies and in clinical trials for staging the severity of Alzheimer's Disease" (Morris, 1993, p. 2412).

PSYCHOMETRIC PROPERTIES: Hughes, Berg, Danziger, Coben, and Martin (1982) reported a study about the development of the CDR as a global measure of dementia (p. 566). Subjects with mild to severe dementia and healthy controls were rated for cognitive function with the CDR and tested with other measures of impairment. CDR ratings were correlated ($p <$ 0.0001) with scores for the Blessed Dementia Scale (0.74; see entry in this book), the Short Portable Mental Status Questionnaire (0.84; Pfeiffer, 1975), and the Face Hand Test (0.57; Fink, Green, & Bender, 1952). In pilot testing, interrater reliability for the instrument was 0.89 (Hughes et al., 1982, p. 569). Five physicians rated videotaped assessment interviews conducted by physicians and recorded for later independent review. There was 80% agreement for the overall CDRs and a range of agreement for scores in the six categories between 68% and 88% (Burke, Miller, Rubin, & Boland, 1988). Three clinical nurse specialists using the same methodology achieved similar levels of reliability for CDR ratings between nurses (81%) and between physicians and nurses (80%). Range of agreement for the six categories between nurses was 73% to 81% and between MDs and nurses was 74% to 83% (McCulla et al., 1989). Kappa statistics computed for agreement in the two reliability studies were interpreted as being in the good to excellent range (0.58 to 0.85).

PROCEDURE: The CDR is completed in a semistructured interview with a patient and an appropriate informant. The printed tool has a 5×6 box graphic format. Phrases describing impairment are printed in a 5-point scale (rows) for each of the six categories (columns). The box most applicable to the person being rated is checked for each category. Impairment is rated as "decline from the person's usual level due to cognitive loss alone, not impairment due to other factors such as physical handicap or depression" (Morris, 1993, p. 2413). If raters make observations leading to ambiguous ratings, with two boxes in a category applying to the subject, the rule is to check the box for greater impairment.

SAMPLE ITEM:

Memory category:		
0	None	No memory loss or slight inconsistent forgetfulness
0.5	Questionable	Consistent slight forgetfulness; partial recollection of events; "benign" forgetfulness
1	Mild	Moderate memory loss; more marked for recent events; defect interferes with everyday activities
2	Moderate	Severe memory loss; only highly learned material retained; new material rapidly lost
3	Severe	Severe memory loss; only fragments remain

(Morris, 1993, p. 2413)

SCORING: The CDR has a 5-point scale: *none* (0), *questionable* (0.5), *mild* (1), *moderate* (2), and *severe* (3). The clinician or researcher may also compute a global CDR rating using detailed clinical scoring rules provided by the authors (Morris, 1993, p. 2413).

SOURCE: A copy of the latest version of the instrument and the scoring rules are presented in Morris (1993). The publishers of *Neurology* hold the copyright.

REFERENCES

Berg, L. (1988). Clinical Dementia Rating (CDR). *Psychopharmacology Bulletin, 24,* 637-639.

Burke, W. J., Miller, J. P., Rubin, E., & Boland, S. (1988). Reliability of the Washington University Clinical Dementia Rating (CDR). *Archives of Neurology, 45,* 31-32.

Fink, M., Green, M. A., & Bender, M. B. (1952). The Face-Hand Test as a diagnostic sign of organic mental syndrome. *Neurology, 2,* 46-58.

Hughes, C. P., Berg, L., Danziger, W. L., Coben, L., & Martin, R. L. (1982). A new clinical scale for the staging of dementia. *British Journal of Psychiatry, 140,* 566-572.

McCulla, M. M., Coats, M., Van Fleet, N., Duchek, J., Grant, E., & Morris, J. C. (1989). Reliability of clinical nurse specialists in staging of dementia. *Archives of Neurology, 46,* 1210-1211.

Morris, J. C. (1993). The Clinical Dementia Rating (CDR): Current version and scoring rules. *Neurology, 43,* 2412-2414.

Pfeiffer, E. (1975). A short portable mental status questionnaire for the assessment of organic brain deficit in elderly patients. *Journal of the American Geriatrics Society, 23,* 433-441.

CLOCK TEST

AUTHORS: H. Tuokko, A. Horton, and T. Hadjistavropoulos
ADDRESS: H. Tuokko, PhD
            Clinic for Alzheimer's Disease and Related Disorders
            University Hospital, University of British Columbia Site
            2211 Wesbrook Mall
            Vancouver, BC V6T 2B5, Canada

DESCRIPTION: The Clock Test (Tuokko, Hadjistavropoulos, Miller, & Beattie, 1992) has three components: clock drawing, clock setting, and clock reading. It is a screening and research tool for cognitive impairment, particularly Alzheimer's disease (AD), with a refined scoring system to measure clock-drawing performance both quantitatively and qualitatively.

PSYCHOMETRIC PROPERTIES: There is a relationship between clock drawing and cognitive status (Shulman, Shedletsky, & Silver, 1986; Sunderland et al., 1989). The clock-drawing performance of 30 AD patients was judged independently by three raters; reliability coefficients ranged between 0.90 and 0.95. For a different 32-patient sample, tested at a 4-day interval, the test-retest reliability coefficient was 0.70. Significant differences in scores for normal elderly ($n = 62$) and AD patients ($n = 58$) were found for drawing errors, correct settings, and correct readings (Tuokko et al., 1992).

PROCEDURE: For clock drawing, the subject is first asked to imagine that a predrawn circle is a clock and to place numbers on the face appropriately. Second, the subject is asked to draw hands on the clock face to indicate "10 past 11." For clock setting, circles with marks (no numbers) are introduced, and the subject is asked to draw hands on the clock that will indicate specific times. For clock reading, five separate circles are presented with the same marks (no numbers) and clock hands, indicating the same hours and minutes as for the clock-setting condition, but in a different order.

SAMPLE ITEMS: For the clock setting and clock reading, settings tested are "1) one o'clock, 2) ten past eleven, 3) three o'clock, 4) nine-fifteen, and 5) seven-thirty" (Tuokko et al., 1992, p. 580).

SCORING: For clock drawing, errors are scored within the categories: omissions, perseverations, rotations, misplacements, distortions, substitutions, and additions. For clock setting, score 1 point for correct placement of each hand and 1 point for correct lengths of hands (maximum = 3). For clock reading, score 1 point for each hand read correctly and 1 additional point if both are read correctly (maximum = 3).

SOURCE: A manual (Tuokko, Horton, & Hadjistavropoulos, 1990) is available from the authors.

REFERENCES

Shulman, K., Shedletsky, R., & Silver, I. L. (1986). The challenge of time: Clock drawing and cognitive functioning in the elderly. *International Journal of Geriatric Psychiatry, 1,* 135-140.

Sunderland, T., Hill, J. L., Mellow, A. M., Lawlor, B. A., Gundersheimer, J., Newhouse, P. A., & Grafman, J. H. (1989). Clock drawing in Alzheimer's disease: A novel measure of dementia severity. *Journal of the American Geriatrics Society, 37,* 725-729.

Tuokko, H., Hadjistavropoulos, T., Miller, A., & Beattie, L. (1992). The Clock Test: A sensitive measure to differentiate normal elderly from those with Alzheimer disease. *Journal of the American Geriatrics Society, 40,* 579-584.

Tuokko, H., Horton, A., & Hadjistavropoulos, T. (1990). *The Clock Test: Manual for administration and scoring.* (Available from the authors at address listed above)

COGNITIVE ABILITIES SCREENING INSTRUMENT (CASI)

AUTHORS: Evelyn L. Teng, Kazuo Hasegawa, Akira Homma,
            Yukimuchi Imai, Eric Larson, Amy Graves,
            Keiko Sugimoto, Takenori Yamaguchi, Hideo Sasaki,
            Darryl Chiu, and Lon R. White
ADDRESS: Evelyn L. Teng, PhD
            Department of Neurology (GNH5641)
            University of Southern California School of Medicine
            2025 Zonal Avenue
            Los Angeles, CA 90033

DESCRIPTION: The Cognitive Abilities Screening Instrument (CASI) is a tool used to screen for dementia. Initial testing of CASI, which was designed for cross-cultural use in epidemiological studies, took place in Japan and the United States. This instrument can also be used "to monitor disease progress, and to provide a profile of impairment among various cognitive domains" (Teng et al., 1994, p. 46). The nine domains addressed by CASI are "attention, concentration/mental manipulation, orientation, short-term memory, long-term memory, language, visual construction, list-generating fluency, abstraction and judgment" (p. 50). The authors suggested that as CASI is adapted for use with different subject groups, items will need to be modified and the tool appropriately coded. For example, the first English prototype intended for "literate English-speaking subjects" is labeled *CASI E-1.0*. The "E" represents English and "1.0" stands for the "first unrevised major version" of CASI in English. The first Japanese version is labeled *CASI J-1.0*.

PSYCHOMETRIC PROPERTIES: Items for this tool are "either identical or similar" to those for three other scales: the Mini-Mental State Examination (MMSE) and the Modified Mini-Mental State Examination (3MS; see entries in this book) and the Hasegawa Dementia Screening Scale (HDSS; Hasegawa, 1983). The clinician or researcher can estimate MMSE, 3MS, and HDSS scores from "subsets of the CASI items" (Teng et al., 1994, p. 45). This feature of CASI allows users to rely on the validity of CASI and to draw comparisons with other samples tested with the other instruments.

PROCEDURE: The CASI was piloted at four sites with convenience samples of 443 persons, 208 with dementia. The mean administration time in minutes for pilot testing was 18.2 for dementia patients and 13.7 for normal controls (Teng et al., 1994, p. 48). Performance on the CASI improved with education and declined with age (p. 48). Teng et al. (1994) determined the extent to which each item distinguished dementia patients from controls. At all four sites, those items that assessed "short-term memory, temporal orientation, and list generating fluency were most sensitive," and those assessing "attention, language abilities, and long-term memory of vital personal information [were] least sensitive" (p. 49).

SAMPLE ITEMS: "What is today's date?" "What day of the week is today?" and "What actions would you take if you lost a borrowed umbrella?" (Teng et al., 1994, pp. 55-56).

SCORING: "The range of scores on the majority of the domains is from 0 to 10. The CASI total score has a range between 0 and 100" (Teng et al., 1994, p. 47). Scoring is intricate; the authors have devised a convenient scoring form.

SOURCE: A copy of the instrument and the scoring form is reprinted in the appendix to Teng et al. (1994). The tool, its manual, and a videotape about test administration, together with "quizzes to qualify potential users on the administration and scoring of the CASI," are available from CASI Materials, c/o L. White, EDB Program, National Institute on Aging, Gateway Building, Room 3C309, National Institutes of Health, Bethesda, MD 20892.

REFERENCES

Hasegawa, K. (1983). The clinical assessment of dementia in the aged: A dementia screening scale for psychogeriatric patients. In M. Bergener, U. Lehr, E. Lang, & R. Schmitz-Scherzer (Eds.), *Aging in the eighties and beyond* (pp. 207-218). New York: Springer.

Teng, E. L., Hasegawa, K., Homma, A., Imai, Y., Larson, E., Graves, A., Sugimoto, K., Yamaguchi, T., Sasaki, H., Chiu, D., & White, L. R. (1994). The Cognitive Abilities Screening Test (CASI): A practical test for cross-cultural epidemiological studies of dementia. *International Psychogeriatrics, 6*(1), 45-58.

COGNITIVE CAPACITY SCREENING EXAMINATION (CCSE)

AUTHORS: John W. Jacobs, David M. Kaufman, and colleagues
ADDRESS: David M. Kaufman, MD
                Montefiore Medical Center
                111 East 210 Street
                Bronx, NY 10467-2490

DESCRIPTION: The Cognitive Capacity Screening Examination (CCSE) is a brief 30-item objective test to screen for the presence or absence of cognitive deficits. The exam was developed by a team of liaison psychiatrists concerned about failure on the part of "house officers" consistently to identify diffuse organic mental syndrome in patients on medical wards.

PSYCHOMETRIC PROPERTIES: Jacobs, Bernhard, Delgado, and Strain (1977) tested the CCSE with four separate samples of medical and psychiatric patients, and hospital staff (Total $N = 135$). The tool was administered independently and consecutively by three observers whose identical scores for six patients were in perfect agreement. Validity was supported by comparisons between CCSE scores and findings from expert psychiatric consultations. There was also a strong association between low scores on the CCSE and diffuse electroencephalograph abnormalities. Even severely anxious and depressed persons scored above 20 on the CCSE. Some scores were lower than the assigned 19 cutoff, however, when subjects had minimal education or poor English language comprehension.

Foreman (1987) compared the CCSE with other measures of cognitive status used with elderly patients. He found that the CCSE was "the most valid and reliable measure of mental status" (p. 219). He pointed out, however, that the 30-item format might place a burden on respondents, thus producing responses that were not valid or reliable. Foreman said that for cognitively intact populations, the CCSE would be the instrument of choice among those that he had reviewed.

PROCEDURE: The CCSE is designed in a one-page format to be used in an interview. It takes 5 to 15 minutes to administer and is introduced with "I would like to ask you a few questions. Some you will find easy and others may be very hard. Just do your best" (Jacobs et al., 1977, p. 45). The examiner may, if necessary, "urge patient once to complete the task" (p. 45). A correct response is checked in the space provided. Incorrect or unusual responses are recorded by the examiner.

SAMPLE ITEMS: "9 + 3 is _____" and "Beginning with Sunday, say the days of the week backwards" (Jacobs et al., 1977, p. 45).

SCORING: The score is the sum of correct responses. A score of 19 or less suggests organic dysfunction (Jacobs et al., 1977, p. 42).

SOURCE: There are copies of the exam in the appendices to Jacobs et al. (1977) and Kaufman, Weinberger, Strain, and Jacobs (1979).

REFERENCES

Foreman, M. D. (1987). Reliability and validity of mental status questionnaires in elderly hospital patients. *Nursing Research, 36,* 216-220.

Jacobs, J. W., Bernhard, M. R., Delgado, A., & Strain, J. J. (1977). Screening for organic mental syndromes in the medically ill. *Annals of Internal Medicine, 86,* 40-46.

Kaufman, D. M., Weinberger, M., Strain, J. J., & Jacobs, J. W. (1979). Detection of cognitive deficits by a brief mental status examination. *General Hospital Psychiatry, 1,* 247-255.

COHEN-MANSFIELD AGITATION INVENTORY (CMAI)

AUTHOR: Jiska Cohen-Mansfield
ADDRESS: Jiska Cohen-Mansfield, PhD
The Research Institute of the Hebrew Home
    of Greater Washington
6121 Montrose Road
Rockville, MD 20852

DESCRIPTION: The purpose of the Cohen-Mansfield Agitation Inventory (CMAI) is to assess the frequency of agitated behaviors in older persons (Cohen-Mansfield, 1991). *Agitation* is defined by the author as "inappropriate verbal, vocal, or motor activity that is not explained by needs or confusion per se" (Cohen-Mansfield & Billig, 1986, p. 712). Agitated behavior, according to the author's framework, is usually demonstrated in three ways: (a) abusive or aggressive behaviors toward self or others, (b) appropriate behavior with inappropriate frequency, or (c) behavior that is inappropriate according to social standards for the specific situation (Cohen-Mansfield, Marx, & Rosenthal, 1989, p. M77). There are five versions of the CMAI: (a) a 30-item long form of agitated behaviors designed to be rated by a caregiver or completed in an interview, (b) a long form with 30 expanded definitions that provides raters with additional examples of each item, (c) a short form consisting of 14 agitated behavior items to be rated on a 5-point scale, (d) a 38-item form that may be used by caretakers of elders residing in the community, and (e) a disruptiveness form that asks the rater also to appraise the extent to which each of the behaviors rated is disruptive.

PSYCHOMETRIC PROPERTIES: Three factors of agitation have been found for nursing home samples: aggressive behavior, physically nonaggressive behavior, and verbally agitated behavior. Analysis of data from community samples revealed four factors: physically nonaggressive behavior, physically aggressive behavior, verbally nonaggressive behavior, and verbally aggressive behavior. Rates of interrater agreement were calculated for each behavior. Averages for agreement rates have ranged between 0.88 and 0.92. The rate of exact agreement for a short form of the instrument was 0.82.

PROCEDURE: Detailed instructions for interviewers are included in a manual (Cohen-Mansfield, 1991). Each behavior is rated for frequency on a

7-point scale. Responses are rated between 1 for *never* engaging in the behavior and 7 for manifesting the behavior *several times an hour.* The rater refrains from attempting to explain the behavior; rather, he or she rates it only for frequency. Rating requires some judgment. When an inappropriate behavior exhibited by a resident is close to a behavior described in an item, the rater adds the behavior to the category.

SAMPLE ITEMS: "Inappropriate dress or disrobing," "Repetitive sentences or questions," and "Pacing, aimless wandering" (Cohen-Mansfield, 1991, p. 9).

SCORING: The author stated that scores for all of the agitated behaviors cannot be meaningfully summed. Rather, calculation of agitation scores will depend on the circumstances of the clinical practice or research. Results of factor analysis will also vary depending on the population studied (Cohen-Mansfield, 1991).

SOURCE: The tools and manual are available from the author. There is a small fee to cover costs of reproduction and mailing.

REFERENCES

Cohen-Mansfield, J. (1991). *Instruction manual for the Cohen-Mansfield Agitation Inventory (CMAI).* (Available from the author at address listed on p. 59)

Cohen-Mansfield, J., & Billig, N. (1986). Agitated behaviors in the elderly. I. A conceptual review. *Journal of the American Geriatrics Society, 34,* 711-721.

Cohen-Mansfield, J., Marx, M. S., & Rosenthal, A. (1989). A description of agitation in a nursing home. *Journal of Gerontology: Medical Sciences, 44,* M77-M84.

COMPREHENSIVE LEVEL OF CONSCIOUSNESS SCALE (CLOCS)

AUTHORS: Daniel E. Stanczak, James G. White, William D. Gouview, Kurt A. Moehle, Michael Daniel, Thomas Novack, and Charles J. Long

ADDRESS: James G. White III, MD
           Department of Neurosurgery
           University of Tennessee
           956 Court, Room 2A27
           Memphis, TN 38163

DESCRIPTION: The Comprehensive Level of Consciousness Scale (CLOCS) is composed of eight scales for assessment of "posture, eye position at rest, spontaneous eye opening, general motor functioning, abnormal ocular movements, pupillary light reflexes, general responsiveness, and best communicative effort" (Stanczak et al., 1984, p. 956). The CLOCS was developed as an "alternative" to the Glasgow Coma Scale (ACS; see entry in this book) that would "assess a wider range of behavior related to impaired consciousness" (p. 955) and would be sensitive to "subtle changes in the patient's condition" (p. 959).

PSYCHOMETRIC PROPERTIES: The properties of the CLOCS were compared with those of the GCS in a study of 101 neurosurgical patients with "impaired consciousness" (Stanczak et al., 1984). Most patients had sustained closed head injuries or cerebrovascular accidents. Reliability and validity coefficients for the two tests were comparable with this sample. Alpha coefficient for the CLOCS was 0.86, test-retest reliability was 0.89, and interrater reliability was 0.96. To estimate validity, nurses rated levels of consciousness ($N = 100$) on a scale of 0 to 6; these ratings were correlated with CLOCS scores (0.71).

PROCEDURE: Each of the eight scales of the CLOCS is preceded by specific instructions. The scale includes a glossary of technical terms related to assessments. Administration takes 3 to 5 minutes once the observer becomes familiar with the scale (Stanczak et al., 1984, p. 959).

SAMPLE ITEM: Scale 6. Pupillary Light Reflexes.

(Instructions: Pupillary reactivity to a strong light source should be noted, and the number of the most appropriate description should be recorded.)

---

7 Normal direct and consensual light reflexes
6 Unilateral absence of direct light reflex
5 Unilateral absence of direct and consensual light reflexes
4 Bilateral absence of direct and consensual light reflexes
3 Hippus [defined in the scale glossary]
2 Pontine (pinpoint) pupils
1 Eyes at midposition, 4-5 mm in diameter, and fixed to all stimuli OR pupils may be slightly irregular and/or slightly unequal
0 Wide pupillary dilation and fixed to all stimuli OR bilateral small (pinpoint) pupils which are fixed to all stimuli

---

(Stanczak et al., 1984, p. 956)

SCORING: The observer records the number of an applicable description on the scale. A total score on the CLOCS may range between 0 and 48.

SOURCE: The CLOCS is reproduced on a single page in Stanczak et al. (1984).

REFERENCE

Stanczak, D. E., White, J. G., Gouview, W. D., Moehle, K. A., Daniel, M., Novack, T., & Long, C. J. (1984). Assessment of level of consciousness following severe neurological insult: A comparison of the psychometric qualities of the Glasgow Coma Scale and the Comprehensive Level of Consciousness Scale. *Journal of Neurosurgery, 60,* 955-960.

CONFUSION ASSESSMENT METHOD (CAM)

AUTHORS: Sharon K. Inouye, Christopher H. van Dyke,
            Cathy A. Alessi, Sharyl Balkin, Alan P. Siegal,
            and Ralph I. Horwitz
ADDRESS: Sharon K. Inouye, MD, MPH
            Yale-New Haven Hospital
            20 York Street, Tompkins Basement 15
            New Haven, CT 06504

DESCRIPTION: The Confusion Assessment Method (CAM) was developed to facilitate quick and accurate identification of delirium by "nonpsychiatrically trained clinicians" (Inouye et al., 1990, p. 941). The instrument was adapted from the revised third edition of the *Diagnostic and Statistical Manual of Mental Disorders* (*DSM-III-R;* American Psychiatric Association, 1987). The authors constructed a CAM questionnaire and rating system to be completed by a clinical evaluator. The CAM identifies and defines "important clinical features of delirium" (Inouye et al., 1990, p. 942). The features are "acute onset and fluctuating course, inattention, disorganized thinking, altered level of consciousness, disorientation, memory impairment, perceptual disturbances, increased or decreased activity, and disturbance of the sleep-wake cycle" (p. 942). The authors also designed a scoring algorithm for diagnosing delirium. Four of the clinical features—(a) acute onset and fluctuating course, (b) inattention, (c) disorganized thinking, and (d) altered level of consciousness—are used in the algorithm. "The diagnosis of delirium requires the presence of features 1 and 2 and either 3 or 4" (p. 942). The CAM has been widely used and translated into three languages.

PSYCHOMETRIC PROPERTIES: The CAM has face validity. The clinical features of the CAM are also the cardinal elements of delirium according to DSM-III-R criteria (Inouye et al., 1990, p. 942). An expert panel of geriatricians, psychiatrists, and neurologists "agreed that each item assessed the feature of delirium that it was intended to assess and that the overall instrument would suitably assess patients with delirium" (p. 943). One concern of the expert panel was whether the CAM could differentiate between dementia and delirium. Concurrent validity was estimated by comparing CAM ratings gathered by geriatricians with psychiatrists' diagnoses of individuals in "two clinically distinct samples" in New Haven ($n = 30$) and Chicago ($n = 26$). The samples were not representative and were selected purposefully to "challenge" the CAM by including patients with dementia and depression (p. 942). Assessments for the psychiatric diagnoses and CAM ratings were conducted independently. Data arranged in a 2×2 table for positive/negative diagnosis by delirium/no delirium showed that 3 of the 56 patients had been misclassified. For the two samples, these figures translated to sensitivity ranging between 94% and 100% and specificity between 90% and 95%. CAM ratings were compared with Mini-Mental State Examination (MMSE; see entry in this book) scores (kappa = 0.64), visual analogue scale ratings for confusion (kappa = 0.82), and other tests. To estimate reliability, a pair of observers simultaneously assessed 10 randomly chosen patients who were interviewed by one of the pair. For presence or absence of delirium, agreement was 100%; for rating all nine clinical features, agreement was 88%, with kappa at 0.67; for assessing the four features needed to complete the algorithm, agreement was 93%, with kappa at 0.81 (p. 944).

PROCEDURE: The CAM instrument was validated for use in a brief structured interview that included the MMSE. It was reported to have been "well understood by physicians, nurses and trained lay interviewers" (Inouye et al., 1990, p. 944). In the validation study, evaluators conducted interviews averaging 20 minutes in length. The CAM questionnaire has detailed questions for the evaluator to answer about each of the nine assessment features. Data are also gathered as needed from family members, caregivers, staff members, or records.

SAMPLE ITEM: Inattention.

Did the patient have difficulty focusing attention, for example, being easily distractible, or having difficulty keeping track of what was being said?

— Not present at any time during the interview.
— Present at some time during interview, but in mild form.
— Present at some time during interview, but in marked form.
— Uncertain. (Inouye et al., 1990, p. 946)

SCORING: Delirium is scored present (1) or absent (0), based on criteria outlined in Inouye (1991).

SOURCE: The CAM questionnaire and its diagnostic algorithm appear in Tables 1 and 2 of the appendix to Inouye et al. (1990). Long and short forms of the questionnaire and a training manual and coding guide (Inouye, 1991) are available from the author.

REFERENCES

American Psychiatric Association. (1987). *Diagnostic and statistical manual of mental disorders* (3rd ed., Rev.). Washington, DC: Author.

Inouye, S. K. (1991). *The Confusion Assessment Method (CAM): Training manual and coding guide.* (Available from the author at address listed above.)

Inouye, S. K., van Dyke, C. H., Alessi, C. A., Balkin, S., Siegal, A. P., & Horwitz, R. I. (1990). Clarifying confusion: The confusion assessment method. *Annals of Internal Medicine, 113,* 941-948.

CORNELL SCALE FOR DEPRESSION IN DEMENTIA (CSDD)

AUTHORS: George S. Alexopoulos, Robert C. Abrams,
            Robert C. Young, and Charles A. Shamoian
ADDRESS: George S. Alexopoulos
            Department of Psychiatry
            The New York Hospital-Westchester Division
            21 Bloomingdale Road
            White Plains, NY 10605

DESCRIPTION: The Cornell Scale for Depression in Dementia (CSDD) is a 19-item instrument designed to provide a quantitative rating for symptoms of depression in persons with dementia (Alexopoulos, Abrams, Young, & Shamoian, 1988a). Data to complete the scale are gathered in interviews with the patient and with care providers on the basis of their round-the-clock observations of symptoms. The CSDD, which was not intended as a diagnostic instrument, taps five major areas: mood-related signs, behavioral disturbance, physical signs, cyclic functions, and ideational disturbance.

PSYCHOMETRIC PROPERTIES: Items were selected from the literature and from consultation with experts. Interrater reliability ($N = 26$) was high, and there was no difference in weighted kappa when patients were severely demented (0.62) or less demented (0.63; Alexopoulos et al., 1988a, p. 275). Coefficient alpha for the scale ($N = 48$) was 0.84. Concurrent validity was demonstrated with a significant relationship (0.83) between total scores and a consensus diagnosis reached by two psychiatrists using the Research Diagnostic Criteria (Spitzer, Endicott, & Robins, 1978). CSDD scores differentiated between demented subjects with "no depression, minor, probable major, and definite major depression" (Alexopoulos et al., 1988a, p. 276). When CSDD scores at admission and discharge ($N = 9$) were compared, results showed that the scale was sensitive to change (Alexopoulos et al., 1988a). The instrument was also validated with a sample ($N = 45$) of "non-demented" persons (Alexopoulos, Abrams, Young, & Shamoian, 1988b).

PROCEDURE: Instructions to raters are: "Ratings should be based on symptoms and signs occurring during the week prior to interview. No score should be given if symptoms result from physical disability or illness" (Alexopoulos et al., 1988a, p. 281). Each item is rated a (*unable to evaluate*), 0 (*absent*), 1 (*mild or intermittent*), or 2 (*severe*).

SAMPLE ITEMS: "Poor self-esteem—self-blame, self-depreciation, feelings of failure" and "Multiple physical complaints (score 0 if GI symptoms only)" (Alexopoulos et al., 1988a, p. 282).

SCORING: Total Cornell Scale scores are sums of item scores.

SOURCE: The instrument appears in the appendices to Alexopoulos et al. (1988a, 1988b).

REFERENCES

Alexopoulos, G. S., Abrams, R. C., Young, R. C., & Shamoian, C. A. (1988a). Cornell Scale for Depression in Dementia. *Biological Psychiatry, 23,* 271-284.

Alexopoulos, G. S., Abrams, R. C., Young, R. C., & Shamoian, C. A. (1988b). Use of the Cornell scale in non-demented patients. *Journal of the American Geriatrics Society, 36,* 230-236.

Spitzer, R., Endicott, J., & Robins, E. (1978). Research diagnostic criteria. *Archives of General Psychiatry, 35,* 773-782.

CRICHTON ROYAL BEHAVIOURAL RATING SCALE (CRBRS) AND CONFUSION RATING (CR)

AUTHORS: R. A. Robinson, A. Charlesworth, and David Wilkin

ADDRESS: Professor David Wilkin
            National Primary Care Research and Development Center
            The University of Manchester
            Oxford Road
            Manchester M13 9PL, United Kingdom

DESCRIPTION: The current version of the Crichton Royal Behavioural Rating Scale (CRBRS) provides estimates of dependency and confusion. It is intended "for use with elderly people in residential or long-stay hospital care" (Wilkin & Thompson, 1989, p. 15). Scores depict "a simple picture of the types of problems encountered, a means of comparing different populations and examining changes in the same population over time" (p. 15). Areas covered are mobility, memory, orientation, communication, cooperation, restlessness, dressing, feeding, bathing, and continence. The Confusion Rating (CR), a subscale of the CRBRS, refers to the areas of memory, orientation, and communication. The CR may be used independently for the purpose of rapid screening for dementia (Vardon & Blessed, 1986, p. 143).

PSYCHOMETRIC PROPERTIES: Estimates of validity have been made by comparing CRBRS scores with independent clinical assessments and contrasting scores for known groups. Total scores of 10 or more were "associated with a diagnosis of psychiatric disorder" (Wilkin & Thompson, 1989, p. 17). Total CRBRS scores were also correlated with "the amount of time spent on the provision of physical care" (p. 17). Scores on the CR were correlated

(–0.82) with scores on the Blessed Information-Memory-Concentration Test (p. 17; see entry in this book). Vardon and Blessed (1986) used the CR to test a stratified random sample ($N = 99$) of elders (22 men, 77 women) living in diverse housing in the United Kingdom. Persons with dementia ($n = 49$) had "significantly higher" CR scores ($t = 3.97$, $p < 0.001$) than other elders, and CR scores for residents of homes for the mentally ill infirmed were significantly higher ($t = 3.45$, $p < 0.001$) than scores for residents in other locations (p. 141). Wilkin and Thompson (1989) reported interrater reliability for the scale at 0.9 and interinformant reliability at 0.95. The number of ratings used to calculate the reliability was not specified, however, and the authors suggested that although the CRBRS was originally developed to guide assessment of individuals, the scale is not sensitive to change in individuals over time (p. 17).

PROCEDURE: There are two forms for the CRBRS. One is an interviewer-administered schedule. The rater "is able to formulate questions appropriate to the individual and the situation, using guidance notes provided" (Wilkin & Thompson, 1989, p. 18). Before proceeding, the examiner prepares by being fully familiar with the notes. Information to complete the scale is gathered, in the context of an unstructured interview, from a third person or persons very familiar with the subject. The interviewer uses probes "to elicit examples of behavior rather than simply accepting the respondent's assessment of the elderly person" (p. 16). The general rule is that ratings are based on actual behaviors, rather than on potential capacities. "An experienced interviewer using the CRBRS can rate 20 persons in an hour" (p. 16). The other form, a self-administered questionnaire, may be used when a more structured approach is needed.

SAMPLE ITEM: Memory Item and Notes, Interviewer-Administered Form:

> 0 = *Complete.* Not at all forgetful or only within a range of normal expectations.
> 1 = *Occasionally forgetful.* Forgets that he or she has done something or forgets where things have been left (e.g., forgets that he collected pension or that she had a bath—tendency to mislay personal possessions), but can easily be reminded and retains awareness of what happened yesterday or last week.
> 2 = *Short-term loss.* Little idea of what happened yesterday or last week but retains memory of more distant past. Can talk sensibly about past, not just isolated incidents.

3 = *Short- and long-term loss.* No memory or only remembers isolated events which may be confused with events that took place at a different time. (Wilkin & Thompson, 1989, p. 20)

SCORING: Except for the memory and feeding items, which are scored from 0 to 3, item scores range from 0 to 4. The sum of item scores is the total CRBRS score. The CR is the sum of scores for memory, orientation, and communication. The CRBRS scores are ordinal; the authors noted that scores of 10 do not imply twice as much dependency as scores of 5. Neither are two individuals, scoring 10, equally dependent, because scores may derive from different dimensions of the measure (p. 18). The CR deals with a single dimension, however, and cutoff scores have been developed from experience with the rating: 0 to 1 = *lucid,* 2 to 3 = *intermediate,* 4 to 6 = *moderately confused,* and 7 to 11 = *severely confused* (Wilkin & Thompson, 1989, p. 15).

SOURCE: Both forms of the CRBRS appear in Wilkin and Thompson (1989). The items for the CR are reprinted in the appendix to Vardon and Blessed (1986).

REFERENCES

Vardon, V. M., & Blessed, G. (1986). Confusion Ratings and Abbreviated Mental Test performance: A comparison. *Age and Ageing, 15,* 139-144.

Wilkin, D., & Thompson, C. (1989). *Users' guide to dependency measures for elderly people.* Sheffield, UK: Sheffield University, Joint Unit of Social Services Research. (Available from Tim Booth, Editor, Department of Sociological Studies, Sheffield University, Western Bank, Sheffield, S10 2TN UK)

DEATH ANXIETY SCALE (DAS)

AUTHOR: Donald I. Templer
ADDRESS: Donald I. Templer, PhD
             Professor of Psychology
             California School of Professional Psychology
             1350 M Street
             Fresno, CA 93721-1881

DESCRIPTION: The Death Anxiety Scale (DAS) is an instrument for measuring death fear or death anxiety, terms the author used synonymously (Lester & Templer, 1992-1993, p. 241). The scale has 15 items with a true-false response format. It was designed for the general population (Templer, 1970, p. 167).

PSYCHOMETRIC PROPERTIES: Seven judges rated 40 items, selected by the author "on a rational basis" (p. 166), for the degree of their association with death anxiety. The 15 items selected for the DAS had the highest average ratings. Test-retest reliability was estimated ($n = 37$) at a 3-week interval ($r = 0.83$), and internal consistency was demonstrated ($n = 31$) with Kuder Richardson Formula 20 at 0.76. The DAS was validated by comparing the DAS scores of psychiatric patients known to have spontaneously verbalized fear or preoccupation with death with scores of a psychiatric patient control group matched for diagnosis, gender, and approximate age. The ages of persons in the sample ranged between 21 and 74. High-anxiety subjects ($n = 21$) had a mean DAS score of 11.62; the control group mean was 6.77. The difference between groups was significant (p. 169). Among two groups of college students ($n = 40$; $n = 48$) who performed a word association task, those with high DAS scores "tended to give words that described emotions" (p. 171). The author also correlated DAS scores with scores on a similar fear of death measure (0.74). Death anxiety scores for elderly persons were reported as tending to be somewhat lower than those for young and middle-aged persons (Lester & Templer, 1992-1993, p. 245).

Templer used similar methods to develop the Death Depression Scale (DDS). The two scales "represent partially distinct entities rather than redundant concepts" (Lester & Templer, 1992-1993, p. 250). Alvarado, Templer, Bresler, and Thomas-Dobson (1992, 1993) suggested that the two scales "and the factors based upon their combined thirty-two items" (p. 118) may be used in research.

PROCEDURE: The scale may be administered orally or as a paper-and-pencil test.

SAMPLE ITEMS: "I am very much afraid to die," "I am not at all afraid to die," and "I am often distressed by the way time flies so rapidly" (Templer, 1970, p. 167).

SCORING: Items are keyed true or false for high death anxiety. Nine items are keyed true and six false. One point is scored for each answer corresponding to the key. McMordie (1979) proposed a Likert format for the scale.

SOURCE: The scale and its key are printed in Templer (1970).

REFERENCES

Alvarado, K. A., Templer, D. I., Bresler, C., & Thomas-Dobson, S. (1993). Are death anxiety and death depression distinct entities? *Omega, 26,* 113-118.
Lester, D., & Templer, D. (1993). Death anxiety scales: A dialogue. *Omega, 26,* 239-253.
McMordie, W. R. (1979). Improving measurement of death anxiety. *Psychological Reports, 44,* 975-980.
Templer, D. I. (1970). The construction and validation of a death anxiety scale. *Journal of General Psychology, 82,* 165-177.

DEMENTIA MOOD ASSESSMENT SCALE (DMAS)

AUTHORS: Trey Sunderland and colleagues at the National Institute
              of Mental Health
ADDRESS: Dr. Trey Sunderland
              Laboratory of Clinical Science
              National Institute of Mental Health
              Bldg. 10, Room 3D/41
              Bethesda, MD 20892-1264

DESCRIPTION: The Dementia Mood Assessment Scale (DMAS) is a 24-item instrument designed to measure the degree of depressed mood in persons with cognitive impairment. It is not intended as a diagnostic instrument. Two scores are derived from the DMAS: the DMAS17 mood scale and the DMAS18-24 severity of dementia scale. The authors stated that the "scale may not be appropriate for more severely demented or uncooperative patients" (Sunderland, Hill, Lawlor, & Molchan, 1988, p. 749).

PSYCHOMETRIC PROPERTIES: Reliability and validity for the DMAS were initially established in work with a sample of 21 persons with mild to moderate dementia. A 20- to 30-minute interview with the subject was simultaneously, but unobtrusively, observed by members of the treatment team. Each subject was independently rated by from 4 to 12 observers. Subjects were also rated by observers using the *NIMH Global Guidelines* (NIMH, 1988) to measure depression, mania, anxiety, psychosis, cognitive impairment, functional impairment, sadness, and anger. There were high percentages of agreement between DMAS and global ratings, with no differences found between experienced and inexperienced raters. DMAS scores were significantly correlated with global ratings for depression and sadness. The results of factor analysis with another sample ($N = 54$) were a four-factor structure explaining 70% of the variance. The factors were labeled Depression, Social Interaction, Anxiety, and Vegetative Symptoms. Associations between scores for global measures and scores for items grouped in the selected factors supported construct validity and confirmed the independence of the subscales (Sunderland, Alterman, et al., 1988).

PROCEDURE: The instrument was designed to be completed for a particular time period, usually a week. Assessment is based on a clinical interview by a trained rater who has had the opportunity to gather objective information from a family member or professional staff member caring for the subject.

SAMPLE ITEM: Depressed Appearance.

 0 = Does not appear depressed *and* denies such when questioned directly.
 2 = Occasionally seems sad and downcast. May admit to "spirits" being low from time to time.
 4 = Frequently appears depressed, irrespective of ability to express or explain underlying thoughts.
 6 = Shows mostly depressed appearance, even to casual observer. May be associated with frequent crying. (Sunderland, Hill, et al., 1988, p. 751)

SCORING: For each of the 24 items, there are four descriptors that the observer rates on a continuum between 0 (*within normal limits*) and 6 (*most severe*). When the subject's behavior falls between descriptors, the item is rated with the odd numbers 1, 3, or 5. The sum of the first 17 items is the score for DMAS17; the sum of Items 18 through 24 is the DMAS18-24 score. There are specific instructions for scoring Items 2, 18, and 19 that the rater will need to read in Sunderland, Hill, et al. (1988).

SOURCE: The instrument is available from the authors. It is also reprinted in Sunderland, Hill, et al. (1988).

REFERENCES

National Institute of Mental Health. (1988). *NIMH Global Guidelines* (Unit on Geriatric Psychopharmacology, Laboratory of Clinical Science). Bethesda, MD: Author.

Sunderland, T., Alterman, I. S., Yount, D., Hill, J. L., Tariot, P. N., Newhouse, P. A., Mueller, E. A., Mellow, A. M., & Cohen, R. M. (1988). A new scale for the assessment of depressed mood in demented patients. *American Journal of Psychiatry, 145,* 955-959.

Sunderland, T., Hill, J. L., Lawlor, B. A., & Molchan, S. E. (1988). NIMH Dementia Mood Assessment Scale (DMAS). *Psychopharmacology Bulletin, 24,* 747-753.

DEPRESSION STATUS INVENTORY (DSI)

AUTHOR: William W. K. Zung
ADDRESS: Elizabeth Marsh Zung
            1816 Woodburn Road
            Durham, NC 27705

DESCRIPTION: The Depression Status Inventory (DSI) is a 20-item, semi-structured, interviewer-rated instrument for "measuring depression as a psychiatric disorder" (Zung, 1976, p. 176). It was developed to be used as an "adjunct" to Zung's Self-Rating Depression Scale (SDS; Zung, 1965), which has the same diagnostic criteria (Zung, 1972). The scale is designed to be used in an interview, and its format includes interview guidelines. However, Zung intended the interviewer to have the "flexibility of modifying the questions and probing for details," to make possible "a smooth interview that does not sound like a question and answer examination" (Zung, 1972, p. 541).

PSYCHOMETRIC PROPERTIES: The author initially used the instrument with consecutively admitted male psychiatric inpatients aged 22 to 75 ($n = 152$), and male and female outpatients aged 14 to 72 ($n = 73$). He reported higher mean DSI scores for patients with depression ($n = 96$) than for patients in five other diagnostic groups ($n = 113$). DSI scores were correlated with SDS scores at 0.87. Reliability was tested with split-half correlations for the

10 even-numbered (0.81) and 10 odd-numbered (0.73) items (Zung, 1972, p. 543).

PROCEDURE: To standardize responses, the interviewer sets a 1-week time context for information gathered with the DSI. Therefore, at least some questions are prefaced with the phrase, "During the past week, have you . . . ?" (Zung, 1972, p. 541). In Zung (1972) and Zung (1976), the author outlined specific rules for making and recording judgments.

SAMPLE ITEMS:

Signs and Symptoms of Depression	Interview Guide for DSI
1. Depressed mood	1. Do you ever feel sad or depressed?
4. Sleep disturbances	4. Frequent and early AM wakings?
7. Decreased libido	7. Do you enjoy looking at, talking or being with attractive men/women?
10. Fatigue	10. How easily do you get tired?

(Zung, 1976, p. 172)

SCORING: Items are scored in terms of intensity, duration, and frequency: 1 = *none or insignificant in intensity or duration, present none or little of the time in frequency,* 2 = *mild in intensity or duration, present some of the time,* 3 = *of moderate severity, present a good part of the time,* and 4 = *severe in intensity or duration, present most or all of the time in frequency* (Zung, 1972, p. 541). Raw DSI scores are converted to Z scores. A conversion chart is provided in Zung (1972, p. 542). Scores below 50 are considered within normal range. Scores between 50 and 59 indicate mild depression, scores between 60 and 69 indicate moderate to severe depression, and scores of 70 or over indicate severe depression (Zung, 1976, p. 177).

SOURCE: The instrument is reprinted in Zung (1972) and in Zung (1976). Mrs. E. M. Zung, who owns the copyright, may be contacted for permission to use the DSI.

REFERENCES

Zung, W. W. K. (1965). A self-rating depression scale. *Archives of General Psychiatry, 12,* 63-70.

Zung, W. W. K. (1972). The Depression Status Inventory: An adjunct to the Self-Rating Depression Scale. *Journal of Clinical Psychology, 28,* 539-543.

Zung, W. W. K. (1976). Depression Status Inventory and Self-Rating Depression Scale. In W. Guy (Ed.), *Early Clinical Drug Evaluation Unit assessment manual for psychopharmacology* (Rev. ed., pp. 172-178, DHEW Pub. No. ADM 76-338). Washington, DC: U.S. Department of Health, Education and Welfare.

DEPRESSIVE SIGNS SCALE (DSS)

AUTHORS: C. L. E. Katona and C. R. Aldridge

ADDRESS: Dr. C. L. E. Katona
St. George's Hospital Medical School
Crammer Terrace
London SW 17 ORE, England

DESCRIPTION: The Depressive Signs Scale (DSS) is a nine-item tool designed to screen for depressive signs in persons diagnosed with dementia (Katona & Aldridge, 1985). When they developed the scale, the authors believed that it was possible "that vulnerability to depression is increased in the presence of dementia as it is in other types of diffuse brain injury" (p. 87). The DSS allows depression to be assessed "without recourse to detection of symptoms by direct questioning of patients" (p. 87).

PSYCHOMETRIC PROPERTIES: Finding no rating scales then available to assess depression in a severely demented population, the authors devised the DSS for their study of the suppression of endogenous cortisol production by dexamethasone with a small sample of patients with dementia ($n = 20$). They also tested a control group of 10 depressed patients with no cognitive defect. Interrater reliability for total scores ranged between 0.94 and 0.99, with weighted kappa for individual items ranging from 0.71 to 1.00. A Mann-Whitney U test showed that DSS scores for the depressed and demented groups were significantly different, $p < 0.05$ (Katona & Aldridge, 1985, p. 85).

PROCEDURE: Items are rated by an observer after a clinical interview with the subject and an interview with the subject's caregiver. Each item has a brief descriptive passage that defines the phenomenon to be measured.

SAMPLE ITEM: "1. *Sad appearance.* Gloom, despair, tearfulness, despondency as suggested by facial expression and posture. Marked = 2, Intermediate = 1, Absent = 0" (Katona & Aldridge, 1985, p. 88).

SCORING: Scores may range from 0 to 17. The range of scores for the authors' sample was 0 to 9 (p. 85).

SOURCE: The scale is printed in Katona and Aldridge (1985).

REFERENCE

Katona, C. L. E., & Aldridge, C. R. (1985). The dexamethasone suppression test and depressive signs in dementia. *Journal of Affective Disorders, 8,* 83-89.

DIRECT ASSESSMENT OF FUNCTIONAL STATUS (DAFS)

AUTHORS: David A. Loewenstein, Ellen Amigo, Ranjan Duara, David Guterman, Deborah Hurwitz, and others
ADDRESS: David A. Loewenstein, PhD
Wien Center for Alzheimer's Disease and
  Memory Disorders
Mount Sinai Medical Center
4300 Alton Road
Miami Beach, FL 33140

DESCRIPTION: The Direct Assessment of Functional Status (DAFS) is a behaviorally based rating system with seven scales: Time Orientation (16 points), Communication Skills (14 points), Transportation (13 points), Financial Skills (21 points), Shopping Skills (16 points), Grooming (14 points), and Eating (10 points; Loewenstein et al., 1989, pp. P120-P121). The DAFS is intended for use with persons living in the community. The authors suggested that the DAFS may be useful when professionals are "asked to judge their patients' ability to handle finances, drive, make basic decisions in the workplace, or live independently" (p. 118).

PSYCHOMETRIC PROPERTIES: Items for the scales were identified from the literature and from clinical experience (Loewenstein et al., 1989, p. P115). The sample participating in the work to validate the instrument were 30 memory-disordered persons with Alzheimer's disease (AD), multiple cerebral infarcts (MCI), or mixed AD and MCI; 11 depressed patients; and 18 normal elderly controls. Interrater reliability was estimated for independent evaluations of memory-disordered patients ($n = 15$; mean age = 75+) and controls ($n = 12$; mean age = 76+); kappas for subscales ranged from 0.91 to 1.0 (p. P116). Test-retest reliability ($n = 26$; mean age = 76+) measured within 3 to 7 weeks showed that significant reliabilities (kappa) ranged from 0.50 to 0.91 for 15 memory-disordered subjects and from 0.77 to 1.0 for 15 normal controls (p. P117). Scores for a task of taking a telephone message were not stable; therefore, it was dropped from the scale. DAFS scores for the patient group ($n = 30$) were correlated with scores on the Blessed Dementia Scale (DS) ($r = -0.58$; see entry in this book), and scores on another format of the DS ($r = -0.67$) modified to tap "functional behavior in the home environment" (p. P117). For the AD patients alone ($n = 11$), correlations with the Blessed tests were –0.65 and –0.68 (p. P118). Validity for the DAFS was supported when ratings for directly observed performance were comparable to independent clinical appraisals of function (range of biserial correlation 0.59 to 0.65). For most scales of the DAFS, scores discriminated between the group of AD patients and other groups of subjects. However, although scores for the AD group were lower for telling time, identifying change, and dressing/grooming, differences were not significant. There were no differences between groups for scores on the eating scale.

PROCEDURE: The procedures for administration are described in Loewenstein et al. (1989).

SAMPLE ITEM: III. Transportation.

(Patient has to correctly identify a driver's correct response to these road signs.) Stop, Yield, One way, No right turn, Green light, Yellow light, Red light, No "U" turn, Railroad crossing, Do not enter, Double yellow line, Passing line, Speed limit. (Loewenstein et al., 1989, p. P121)

SCORING: Depending on the item, the rater scores 1 or 2 points if performance is correct and 0 points if it is incorrect. Scoring codes are printed with the scales.

SOURCE: The DAFS is printed as an appendix to Loewenstein et al. (1989). A manual for administration and scoring the DAFS is available from Dr. Loewenstein.

REFERENCE

Loewenstein, D. A., Amigo, E., Duara, R., Guterman, A., Hurwitz, D., Berkowitz, N., Wilkie, F., Weinberg, G., Black, B., Gittelman, B., & Eisdorfer, C. (1989). A new scale for assessment of functional status in Alzheimer's disease and related disorders. *Journal of Gerontology: Psychological Sciences, 44,* P114-P121.

DISCOMFORT SCALE (DAT-DS)

AUTHORS: Ann C. Hurley, Beverly J. Volicer, Patricia A. Hanrahan, Susan Houde, and Ladislav Volicer

ADDRESS: Ann C. Hurley, RN, DNSc
Geriatric Research, Education, and Clinical Center
Edith Norse Rogers Memorial Veterans Hospital
200 Springs Road
Bedford, MA 01730

DESCRIPTION: The Discomfort Scale, a measure developed from the perspective of nursing personnel practicing with residents in special care Alzheimer's units, was designed to measure discomfort in persons who have lost their verbal abilities to communicate and are at risk for discomfort. The authors believe that discomfort can be observed objectively even in patients who cannot report it verbally. They defined *discomfort* operationally as "the presence of behaviors considered to express a negative emotional and/or physical state that are capable of being observed by a trained rater unfamiliar with the usual behavior pattern of the patient" (Hurley, Volicer, Hanrahan, Houde, & Volicer, 1992, p. 370).

PSYCHOMETRIC PROPERTIES: The scale was developed in three studies. In the first, 26 items were generated empirically in interviews with 45 registered and practical nurses and nursing assistants. Content validity for 18 items (13 positively worded and 5 negatively worded) was established by nine advanced practice nurses. After pilot testing involving independent ratings by two observers using visual analogue scales to determine internal consistency (alpha = 0.77) and test-retest reliability ($r = 0.6$, $p < 0.001$), nine items were retained: (a) noisy breathing, (b) negative vocalization, (c) absence of a look of contentment, (d) looking sad, (e) looking frightened, (f) having a frown, (g) absence of relaxed body posture, (h) looking tense, and (i) fidgeting. In a third 6-month longitudinal study, raters who had been trained with videotapes assessed 82 patients (5 females, 77 males) with advanced Alzheimer's disease (AD), in their natural settings, for frequency, intensity, and duration of behavioral indicators specific for each item. Construct validity was established with detection of differences in discomfort in ratings of AD patients experiencing intermittent illness with fever (Hurley et al., 1992).

PROCEDURE: Raters need to be trained. They review conceptual development of the scale before each rating period, committing the specific behavioral descriptions for each item to memory. To avoid influencing the patient's behavior, they use standard scripts and behaviors. Rating periods are 5 minutes in duration. The rater smiles, introduces him- or herself, and says, "I'll be spending a few minutes with you," then positions him- or herself in such a manner as to be able to hold the patient's wrist to count the pulse rate, hear the patient's noises, and observe his or her facial expressions and the body language of all four extremities.

SAMPLE ITEM: Behavioral indicators for noisy breathing are "negative sounding noise on inspiration or expiration; breathing looks strenuous, labored, or wearing; respirations sound loud, harsh, or gasping; difficulty breathing or trying hard at attempting a good gas exchange; episodic bursts of rapid breaths or hyperventilation" (Hurley et al., 1992, p. 373).

SCORING: Each item is scored one of the following:

Missing data (NA), when the behavior *cannot* be observed. The reason the behavior cannot be observed is provided on the data collection form.

None (0), when the item is *not* observed.

Minimum (1), when at least one description of the item is observed at low intensity for a short time.

Moderate (2) (an exclusion category), when behavior is observed but not at minimum or extreme levels.

Extreme (3), when at least one behavior at high intensity is observed for almost entire rating period, more than one description is present even at low intensity and for short durations, or complete description is observed throughout the rating period.

SOURCE: Scale forms and administrative and scoring procedures are available from the authors.

REFERENCE

Hurley, A. C., Volicer, B. J., Hanrahan, P. A., Houde, S., & Volicer, L. (1992). Assessment of discomfort in advanced Alzheimer patients. *Research in Nursing and Health, 15,* 369-377.

DUKE HEALTH PROFILE (DUKE)

AUTHORS: George R. Parkerson, Jr., W. Eugene Broadhead, and Chiu-Kit J. Tse

ADDRESS: George R. Parkerson, Jr., MD
Department of Community and Family Medicine
Duke University Medical Center
Box 2914
Durham, NC 27710

DESCRIPTION: The Duke Health Profile (DUKE) is a 17-item tool for self-report of health outcomes. It was derived from the 63-item Duke-UNC Health Profile (DUHP; Parkerson et al., 1981). The new scale was designed to be brief, yet still to provide as much essential information as possible (Parkerson, Broadhead, & Tse, 1991, p. 400). Its conceptualization of health conforms with "the three WHO dimensions: physical, mental and social health" (Parkerson, Broadhead, & Tse, 1990, p. 1058). Scores for the DUKE are configured for physical health, mental health, social health, general health, perceived health, self-esteem, anxiety, depression, pain, and disability.

PSYCHOMETRIC PROPERTIES: Face validity for the DUKE is strong. "Each of the 17 items is easy to understand and appears by its wording to measure the aspect of health or dysfunction about which it asks" (Parkerson et al., 1990, p. 1067). Validity and reliability for the DUKE were estimated with data from a secondary analysis of scores for the DUHP ($N = 683$). Alpha coefficients for DUKE scores ranged between 0.55 and 0.78. Spearman rank-order correlations to estimate test-retest reliability ($N = 55$) at 1- to 8-week intervals ranged from 0.30 to 0.78; the lowest coefficients (0.30 and 0.41) were associated with the single-item scores for disability and pain, known to be relatively unstable. Investigations of validity of the DUKE included comparisons made with DUHP scores, sociodemographic variables, scores with other instruments, and type of health problem. The results have supported the authors' hypotheses, leading them to argue for "the usefulness of the DUKE in research, health promotion, and clinical practice" (p. 1067).

PROCEDURE: The DUKE is a one-page paper-and-pencil questionnaire with clear instructions printed at the top of the page. The first seven items do not refer to a specific time frame. The contexts for the other 10 items are either "today" or "the past week." For each item, the respondent chooses from among three possible responses.

SAMPLE ITEMS: "I am happy with my family relationships" ("Yes, describes me exactly," "Somewhat describes me," or "No, doesn't describe me at all") and *"Today* would you have any physical trouble or difficulty: Walking up a flight of stairs?" ("None," "Some," "A lot") (Parkerson et al., 1990, p. 1070).

SCORING: Detailed instructions for deriving the scores from DUKE items appear on the back of each test form.

SOURCE: The instrument is reprinted in the appendix to Parkerson et al. (1990) and Parkerson et al. (1991). Scoring instructions are included in the appendix to Parkerson et al. (1990). The DUKE is copyrighted by the Department of Community and Family Medicine at Duke University Medical Center. Copies of the instrument are available from the authors.

REFERENCES

Parkerson, G. R., Jr., Broadhead, W. E., & Tse, C.-K. J. (1990). The Duke Health Profile: A 17-item measure of health and dysfunction. *Medical Care, 28,* 1056-1072.

Parkerson, G. R., Jr., Broadhead, W. E., & Tse, C.-K. J. (1991). Development of the 17-item Duke Health Profile. *Family Practice, 8,* 396-401.

Parkerson, G. R., Jr., Gehlbach, S. H., Wagner, E. H., James, S. A., Clapp, N. E., & Muhlbaier, L. H. (1981). The Duke-UNC Health Profile: An adult health status instrument for primary care. *Medical Care, 19,* 806-828.

DYSFUNCTIONAL BEHAVIOR RATING INSTRUMENT (DBRI)

AUTHORS: D. W. Molloy, W. E. McIlroy, G. H. Guyatt, and J. A. Lever
ADDRESS: Dr. Willie Molloy, Director
            Geriatric Research Group
            McMaster University, Department of Medicine
            Hamilton Civic Hospitals, Henderson General Division
            711 Concession Street
            Hamilton, Ontario L8V 1C3, Canada

DESCRIPTION: The Dysfunctional Behavior Rating Instrument (DBRI) is a 22-item tool developed to be completed by caregivers. It measures "dysfunctional behavior in cognitively impaired older adults living in the community" (Molloy, McIlroy, Guyatt, & Lever, 1991, p. 103). The authors defined dysfunctional behavior as "an inappropriate action or response, other than an activity of daily living (ADL), in a given social milieu, that is a problem for the caregiver" (p. 103). The tool covers behaviors considered "demanding, acting out, withdrawing, psychotic, paranoid, disruptive, repetitive, or inappropriate" (p. 104).

PSYCHOMETRIC PROPERTIES: Construct validity was supported with significant correlations between DBRI ratings and scores for 184 community-dwelling elders on other measures of behavior. The instrument had test-retest reliability, with an intraclass correlation coefficient of 0.75 ($N = 35$).

PROCEDURE: Caregivers are asked to rate the frequency of behaviors as well as their responses to the behaviors.

SAMPLE ITEMS: "Asked same question over and over," "Was hiding things," and "Kept changing mind" (Molloy, 1991, pp. 371-373).

SCORING: For each item, frequency is rated on a 6-point scale (0 = *never* through 5 = *more than five times a day*), and response is rated on a similar range of choices (0 = *no problem* through 5 = *great deal of problem*). Higher scores indicate greater impairment.

SOURCE: The instrument is printed in Molloy (1991) and is also available from the authors.

REFERENCES

Molloy, D. W. (Ed.). (1991). *Common sense geriatrics.* Boston: Blackwell Scientific Publications.

Molloy, D. W., McIlroy, W. E., Guyatt, G., & Lever, J. A. (1991). Validity and reliability of the Dysfunctional Behavior Rating Scale. *Acta Psychiatrica Scandinavica, 84,* 103-106.

DYSKINESIA IDENTIFICATION SYSTEM CONDENSED USER SCALE (DISCUS)

AUTHORS: Robert L. Sprague and John E. Kalachnik
ADDRESSES: Robert L. Sprague, PhD
University of Illinois
51 Gerty Drive
Champagne, IL 61820

John E. Kalachnik, MEd
Minnesota Department of Human Services
444 Lafayette Road
St. Paul, MN 55155

DESCRIPTION: The Dyskinesia Identification System Condensed User Scale (DISCUS) is a 15-item rating scale, derived from a longer 34-item instrument, the Dyskinesia Identification System-Coldwater (DIS-Co; Sprague et al., 1984). The DISCUS is intended for early detection, monitoring, and assessment of tardive dyskinesia (TD) in developmentally disabled persons, psychiatric patients, and nursing home residents. Training of raters is absolutely necessary to get reliable ratings (Kalachnik & Sprague, 1994; Kalachnik, Sprague, & Slaw, 1988).

PSYCHOMETRIC PROPERTIES: The instrument was initially used with samples of developmentally disabled patients. To test interrater reliability, trained pairs of raters independently assessed 148 subjects simultaneously. The reliability coefficient was 0.92 (Sprague, Kalachnik, & Slaw, 1989, p. 144). Stability was estimated with test-retest scores (0.40; $p < 0.001$) for 128 subjects assessed at a 2-week interval (p. 143). Mentally ill persons ($n = 277$) were also assessed; interrater reliability for total scores was estimated at 0.91 (Sprague & Kalachnik, 1991, p. 55), and coefficients for items ranged from 0.45 to 0.93 (p. 54). To assess validity of the measure, DISCUS scores of a TD group ($n = 108$) were compared with those of a matched no-TD group ($n = 108$); mean scores were significantly different. With reference to physicians' diagnoses, 93.1% of cases ($n = 216$) were classified accurately when "5" was the cutoff score. With data from a large combined sample ($N = 7,507$), the authors found that the percentage of each age group with total DISCUS scores above 5 gradually increased with age (p. 56).

PROCEDURE: Unless they are trained, raters do not have the ability to assess for TD accurately. Standardized 10-hour training workshops and practice with videotapes are recommended. This training should be followed by practice in rating patients, verified for accuracy by comparison with ratings made by experts (Kalachnik et al., 1988). The examination procedure takes from 5 to 15 minutes. Seven areas of the body are assessed: facial, ocular, oral, lingual, head/neck/trunk, upper limb, and lower limb. These areas are observed as the subject performs the prescribed examination tasks. The level of the subject's cooperation is also rated.

SAMPLE ITEM: Chewing/Lip Smacking (scored 0, 1, 2, 3, 4, or NA). DISCUS Item Definition: "4. *Chewing:* circular or up and down jaw movements similar to chewing gum: DO NOT include jaw tremor; and/or *Lip Smacking:* quick parting of the lips which usually produces a smacking sound" (Sprague et al., 1989, pp. 145-146).

SCORING: Items are scored on a 5-point scale from 0 (*not present*) to 4 (*severe*). Definitions for each level of rating are given on the instrument. For example, the 1 or "minimal" rating means that "abnormal movements are difficult to detect *or* movements are easy to detect but occur only once or twice in a short nonrepetitive manner" (Sprague et al., 1989, p. 145).

SOURCE: Copies of the DISCUS, Item Definitions, and the DISCUS Examination Procedure are printed as appendices to Sprague et al. (1989). A copy of the original 34-item DIS-Co, which has been studied by Bostrom and Walker (1990), appears in Sprague et al. (1984). There is information about training raters in Sprague et al. (1984, 1989).

REFERENCES

Bostrom, A. C., & Walker, M. E. (1990). Validation of TD as measured by DIS-Co. *Nursing Research, 39,* 274-279.

Kalachnik, J. E., & Sprague, R. L. (1994). How well do physicians, pharmacists, and psychologists assess tardive dyskinesia movement? *Annals of Pharmacotherapy, 28,* 185-190.

Kalachnik, J. E., Sprague, R. L., & Slaw, K. M. (1988). Training clinical personnel to assess for tardive dyskinesia. *Progress in Neuro-Pharmacological and Biological Psychiatry, 12,* 749-762.

Sprague, R. L., & Kalachnik, J. E. (1991). Reliability, validity, and a total score cut-off for the Dyskinesia Identification System Condensed User Scale (DISCUS) with mentally ill and mentally retarded populations. *Psychopharmacology Bulletin, 27,* 51-58.

Sprague, R. L., Kalachnik, J. E., Breuning, S. E., Davis, V. J., Ullman, R. K., Cullari, S., Davison, N. A., Ferguson, D. G., & Hoffner, B. A. (1984). The Dyskinesia Identification System-Coldwater (DIS-Co): A tardive dyskinesia rating scale for the developmentally disabled. *Psychopharmacology Bulletin, 20,* 328-338.

Sprague, R. L., Kalachnik, J. E., & Slaw, K. M. (1989). Psychometric properties of the Dyskinesia Identification System Condensed User Scale (DISCUS). *Mental Retardation, 27,* 141-148.

ENFORCED SOCIAL DEPENDENCY SCALE (ESDS)

AUTHORS: Ruth McCorkle, Katherine Young, and Jeanne Q. Benoliel
ADDRESS: Ruth McCorkle, PhD, RN, Director
            Center for Advancing Care in Serious Illness
            School of Nursing, University of Pennsylvania
            420 Guardian Drive
            Philadelphia, PA 19104

DESCRIPTION: The Enforced Social Dependency Scale (ESDS) is a 10-item measure of functional status with two subscales: Personal Competence and Social Competence (McCorkle et al., 1994). It was designed for use with persons who have recently experienced an illness such as cancer, stroke, or heart attack. To rate personal competence, the interviewer assesses eating, dressing, walking, traveling, bathing, and toileting. The Social Competence subscale pertains to home, work, social and recreational activities, and behaviors related to communication. The authors defined social dependency as "needing help from other people in order to perform activities or roles that under ordinary circumstances adults can do for themselves" (p. 245).

PSYCHOMETRIC PROPERTIES: Initially, the tool was designed to measure three "capacities" of social dependency: self-care competence, mobility competence, and social competence (Benoliel, McCorkle, & Young, 1980, p. 4). Factor analysis later showed two "unique factors" (Moinpour, McCorkle, & Saunders, 1992, p. 29), and the authors reduced the self-care and mobility competence components to the current subscale for personal competence. Reliability coefficients for segments of the original format ranged from 0.79 to 0.82; for the total scale, the alpha coefficient was 0.90. Interrater reliability was reported at 95% (Benoliel et al., 1980, pp. 7-8). For a study of cancer patients, alpha coefficients for the ESDS ranged between 0.81 and 0.90 (McCorkle et al., 1994, p. 247). In a study to assess the effects of home nursing care on patients with progressive lung cancer, the home nursing care groups were independent, as measured by the ESDS, 6 weeks longer than the comparison office care group (McCorkle et al., 1989, p. 1379). In a study about discharge planning, Naylor (1990) used the ESDS to screen the functional status of 40 hospitalized elders aged 70 and older.

PROCEDURE: Data to complete the ESDS are collected in an interview that takes from 10 to 30 minutes. The interviewer should be familiar with the guide before proceeding. In the initial interview, the observer asks questions from the interview guide to elicit information comparing the current situation with what had been usual for the patient before his or her illness. Responses are recorded in a narrative form, and the observer later converts the narrative information into a score for each item, using definitions from the ESDS coding instructions. The follow-up or ongoing interviewer asks about "the last week."

PARTIAL ITEM:

2. Do you have problems dressing yourself now that you didn't have before your illness (e.g., bending to put on shoes, stretching to pull something over your head); has surgery made it harder to get dressed? (McCorkle, 1988, p. 3)

SCORING: The range for rating personal competence items is 1 to 6, with a range for the personal competence score from 6 to 36. With the exception of the communication item, for which ratings range between 1 and 3, the range of ratings for social competence is 1 to 4. Scores for social competence range between 4 and 15. The total social dependency score is the sum of the scores for personal and social competence and ranges from 10 to 51. Higher scores reflect greater dependency.

SOURCE: The instrument is available from Dr. McCorkle, who holds the copyright. There are separate guides for the initial and ongoing interviews. The user will also need the ESDS coding instructions, which include definitions of terms used for ratings.

REFERENCES

Benoliel, J. Q., McCorkle, R., & Young, K. (1980). Development of a social dependency scale. *Research in Nursing and Health, 3,* 3-10.

McCorkle, R. (1988). *Enforced Social Dependency Scale initial interview guide.* (Available from the authors at address listed above)

McCorkle, R., Benoliel, J. Q., Donaldson, G., Georgiadou, F., Moinpour, C., & Goodell, B. (1989). A randomized clinical trial of home nursing care for lung cancer patients. *Cancer, 64,* 1375-1382.

McCorkle, R., Jepson, C., Malone, D., Lusk, E., Braitman, L., Buhler-Wilkerson, K., & Daly, J. (1994). The impact of posthospital home care on patients with cancer. *Research in Nursing and Health, 17,* 243-251.

Moinpour, C. M., McCorkle, R., & Saunders, J. (1992). Measuring functional status. In M. Frank-Stromborg (Ed.), *Instruments for clinical nursing research* (pp. 23-45). Boston: Jones & Bartlett.

Naylor, M. D. (1990). Comprehensive discharge planning for hospitalized elderly. *Nursing Research, 39,* 156-161.

EPWORTH SLEEPINESS SCALE (ESS)

AUTHOR: Murray W. Johns
ADDRESS: Dr. Murray W. Johns
              Sleep Disorders Unit, Epworth Hospital
              Erin Street
              Richmond, Victoria 3121, Australia

DESCRIPTION: Daytime sleepiness is an indicator of sleep debt in someone who is sleep deprived, as well as a symptom of a sleep disorder (Dement, 1996). The standard method for measuring daytime sleepiness has been the Multiple Sleep Latency Test (MSLT; Carskadon & Dement, 1985), a complex procedure that requires patients to have polysomnographic recordings in sleep laboratories. The Epworth Sleepiness Scale (ESS) is a paper-and-pencil instrument designed to measure an individual's average sleep propensity in daily life (Johns, 1994). The ESS measures a range of sleep propensities from very high to very low in a simple and inexpensive way. Subjects rate themselves on the likelihood that they could doze off or fall asleep in eight different, common, real-life situations. The items for the scale were derived from observations about daytime sleep and sleepiness (Johns, 1991).

PSYCHOMETRIC PROPERTIES: In validation studies, 150 patients with sleep disorders and 30 controls ranging in age from 18 to 78 years responded to the ESS. Twenty-seven of the patients had MSLTs, and 138 had overnight polysomnography. ESS scores of control subjects ranged between 2 and 10, with a mean of 5.9 and a standard deviation of 2.2. ESS scores of 16 or higher, which reflected high levels of daytime sleepiness, were found in patients with moderately severe sleep disorders. The ESS scores distinguished between sleep disorder diagnostic groups known to be associated with different levels of sleepiness on the basis of multiple sleep latency testing (Johns, 1991, p. 543). ESS and MSLT scores were significantly correlated. Eighty-seven "healthy" medical students responded to ESS items and were retested at a 5-month interval. Their mean scores were 7.6 with a standard deviation of 3.8. A t test for the mean difference between their paired scores was not significant, and the coefficient for the Pearson correlation between scores was 0.82 (Johns, 1992, p. 378). Scores for 54 patients with obstructive sleep apnea syndrome were significantly different following treatment with continuous positive airway pressure. The mean difference between pre- and post-treatment scores was 7.0 (p. 378). Alpha coefficients for ESS scores of various groups have ranged from 0.74 to 0.88 (Johns, 1994, p. 708). Factor analysis of scores has shown that the ESS measures one main variable (p. 708). Johns (1991) pointed out that valid use of the scale assumes that subjects are able to recall or estimate whether they have "dozed off during the day as part of their usual way of life in recent times" (p. 544).

PROCEDURE: Subjects are asked, "How likely are you to doze off or fall asleep in the following situations, in contrast to just feeling tired?" (Johns,

1991, p. 541). If subjects have not recently experienced a situation as depicted in an item, they are asked to estimate how the situation would have affected them (Johns, 1991, p. 541). Completion of the ESS takes just a few minutes. Reliable estimates of a partner's dozing behaviors have also been provided by spouses (Johns, 1994, p. 707).

SAMPLE ITEM: "Sitting inactive in a public place (e.g., a theatre or a meeting)" (Johns, 1991, p. 541).

SCORING: For each item, subjects select a response from a 4-point scale: "0 = would *never* doze, 1 = *slight* chance of dozing, 2 = *moderate* chance of dozing, 3 = *high* chance of dozing" (Johns, 1991, p. 541). Total ESS scores range from 0 to 24.

SOURCE: A copy of the instrument appears in Johns (1991).

REFERENCES

Carskadon, M. A., & Dement, W. C. (1985). The Multiple Sleep Latency Test: What does it measure? *Sleep, 5,* S67-S72.

Dement, W. C. (1996). *Sleepwatchers* (2nd ed.). Menlo Park, CA: Nychthemeron.

Johns, M. W. (1991). A new method for measuring daytime sleepiness: The Epworth Sleepiness Scale. *Sleep, 14,* 540-545.

Johns, M. W. (1992). Reliability and factor analysis of the Epworth Sleepiness Scale. *Sleep, 15,* 376-381.

Johns, M. W. (1994). Sleepiness in different situations measured by the Epworth Sleepiness Scale. *Sleep, 17,* 703-710.

EVEN BRIEFER ASSESSMENT SCALE FOR DEPRESSION (EBAS-DEP)

AUTHORS: Nicholas Allen, David Ames, Deborah Ashby, Kerryn
             Bennetts, Virginia Tuckwell, and Christopher West
ADDRESS: Dr. David Ames
             University of Melbourne Department of Psychiatry
             Royal Melbourne Hospital
             Parkville, Victoria 3050, Australia

DESCRIPTION: The Even Briefer Assessment Scale for Depression (EBAS-DEP) is an eight-item instrument for screening depression in late life. It was intended especially for use "in situations where depression is otherwise likely to be missed altogether and where psychiatric opinion can be requested if a high score is found" (Allen et al., 1994, p. 217). Items of the EBAS-DEP reflect cognitive and affective rather than somatic symptoms.

PSYCHOMETRIC PROPERTIES: To derive the EBAS-DEP, the authors analyzed data from 811 older persons, subjects in five studies conducted in London and Melbourne (Allen et al., 1994, p. 213). EBAS items were selected from the original 21-item Depression Scale of the Brief Assessment Scale (BAS-DEP; Mann et al., 1989). Items chosen were those with the highest item-to-total-scale correlations. The BAS-DEP itself had been derived from scales in the Comprehensive Assessment and Referral Evaluation (CARE; Gurland et al., 1977). The shortened EBAS was validated in three ways. The authors assessed the relative performance of the original and shortened versions of the instrument and established the cutoff that "provided the best trade-off between sensitivity and specificity for the data set" (Allen et al., 1994, p. 215). Scores on the EBAS-DEP ($n = 211$) were compared with diagnoses from the third, revised edition of the *Diagnostic and Statistical Manual of Mental Disorders* (American Psychiatric Association, 1987) made by a psychiatrist and with scores from an analysis with AGECAT (Copeland, Dewey, & Griffith-Jones, 1986), a diagnostic computer program (Allen et al., 1994, p. 216). The original BAS-DEP had a "better overall performance" but differences were not statistically significant (Allen et al., 1994, p. 216). EBAS-DEP scores were comparable to diagnoses made by a psychiatrist. The EBAS had high sensitivity at the expense of a lower specificity; that is, a "greater tendency to classify as depressed subjects who are not so according to the long scale" (Allen et al., 1994, p. 216).

PROCEDURE: Raters make judgments about whether eight assessment propositions about the patient are satisfied. Information is gathered in an interview. The time context for the inquiry is 1 month. For each of the eight items, the procedure for the EBAS-DEP requires that the rater ask the specific question "exactly as printed" on the instrument. However, there may be flexibility in follow-up questions "to clarify the initial answer until the rater can make a clear judgement as to whether the proposition is satisfied or not" (Allen et al., 1994, p. 219).

SAMPLE ITEM:

Question	Assessment Proposition
During the past month, have you *ever* felt that life was not worth living?	Has felt that life was not worth living at some time during the past month.

(Allen et al., 1994, p. 219)

SCORING: If the proposition to be assessed is satisfied, the rater scores the item 1; if not, the item is scored 0. A score of 3 or more for the scale "indicates the probable presence of a depressive disorder which may need treatment, and the patient should be assessed in more detail or referred for psychiatric evaluation" (Allen et al., 1994, p. 219).

SOURCE: The instrument is printed in Allen et al. (1994).

REFERENCES

Allen, N., Ames, D., Ashby, D., Bennetts, K., Tuckwell, V., & West, C. (1994). A brief sensitive screening instrument for depression in late life. *Age and Ageing, 23,* 213-218.

American Psychiatric Association. (1987). *Diagnostic and statistical manual of mental disorders* (3rd ed., Rev.). Washington, DC: Author.

Copeland, J. R. M., Dewey, M. E., & Griffith-Jones, H. M. (1986). A computerised psychiatric diagnostic system and case nomenclature for elderly subjects: GMS and AGECAT. *Psychological Medicine, 16,* 89-99.

Gurland, B. J., Kuriansky, J. B., Sharpe, L. K., Simon, R., Stiller, P., & Birkett, P. (1977). The Comprehensive Assessment and Referral Evaluation (CARE): Rationale, development and reliability. *International Journal of Aging and Human Development, 8,* 9-42.

Mann, A. H., Ames, D., Graham, N., Weyerer, S., Eichhorn, S., Platz, S., Snowden, J., Hughes, F., & Ticehurst, S. (1989). The reliability of the Brief Assessment Schedule. *International Journal of Geriatric Psychiatry, 4,* 221-225.

EVERYDAY INDICATORS OF IMPAIRED COGNITION (EIIC)

AUTHORS: Donna L. Algase and Cynthia A. Beel-Bates
ADDRESS: Dr. Donna Algase and Ms. Cynthia A. Beel-Bates
            University of Michigan School of Nursing
            400 North Ingalls Building
            Ann Arbor, MI 48109-2007

DESCRIPTION: The Everyday Indicators of Impaired Cognition (EIIC), a 19-item performance measure, was designed to assess nursing home residents for performance errors in four domains of cognitive functioning: abstract thinking, judgment, language, and spatial skills (Algase & Beel-Bates, 1993). The authors wanted a screening measure that could "lead to more accurate detection, description, and differentiation of acute and chronic cognitive impairments" (p. 57). The advantages of such a tool would be that it could reveal information that "would be useful in designing nursing care to reinforce capabilities while compensating for limitations" (p. 58).

PSYCHOMETRIC PROPERTIES: In their first study, the authors established content validity for the instrument. They asked 10 content experts to rate relevance of items to cognitive impairment and the nursing home context. The content validity index for the EIIC was 1.0 (Algase & Beel-Bates, 1993, p. 60). The authors studied a nursing home sample ($N = 198$) selected with a stratified random cluster approach. After factor analysis, an original 40-item EIIC was reduced to 23 items. Memory and orientation items were deleted. Cronbach's alpha "ranged from 0.77 for the judgment factor to a high of 0.91 for the language items" (p. 61). Item-to-subscale correlations were moderate to high, and intersubscale correlations were appropriately low to moderate. Interrater reliability was not estimated.

PROCEDURE: The scale is brief and easy to administer.

SAMPLE ITEM: "What would you do if you saw a fire here?" (Algase & Beel-Bates, 1990, p. 1).

SCORING: Each error is scored as 1 and each correct response as 0.

SOURCE: Copies of the tool are available from the authors, who own the copyright.

REFERENCES

Algase, D. L., & Beel-Bates, C. A. (1990). *Everyday Indicators of Impaired Cognition.* (Available from the authors at address listed above)

Algase, D. L., & Beel-Bates, C. A. (1993). Everyday Indicators of Impaired Cognition: Development of a new screening scale. *Research in Nursing and Health, 16,* 57-66.

FACES SCALE

AUTHORS: Frank M. Andrews and Stephen B. Withey
ADDRESS: Frank M. Andrews
            Institute for Social Research
            University of Michigan
            Ann Arbor, MI 48106

DESCRIPTION: The Faces Scale is a measure of subjective well-being in a single-item format. The scale has seven stylized faces in which the shape of the mouth varies gradually from a very positive big smile through a neutral straight line to a very negative turned-down expression of the mouth. The scale is particularly useful when there is a need for a graphic rather than a verbal method of measuring perceived well-being. Unlike other single-item measures of well-being, the Faces Scale offers explicitly identifiable categories for the respondent to select.

PSYCHOMETRIC PROPERTIES: Data gathered with the scale in the Andrews and Withey (1976) studies showed median validity coefficients of 0.82. The authors reported that the distributions for data gathered with the scale showed substantial clustering at the positive end.

PROCEDURE: Introduce test by saying something like "In this exercise you will look at some pictures of faces." The subject is shown the pictures. The investigator says, "Here are some faces. They are expressing various feelings. Under each face there is a letter." Then, depending on clinical or research plan, he or she asks something like "Which face comes closest to expressing how you feel about [your life as a whole]?"

SCORING: Faces are lettered A, B, C, D, E, F, and G.

   A = 1, B = 2, C = 3, D = 4, E = 5, F = 6, and G = 7.

SOURCE: The scale is printed in Andrews and Withey (1976) and Andrews and Robinson (1991).

REFERENCES

Andrews, F. M., & Robinson, J. P. (1991). Measures of subjective well-being. In J. P. Robinson, P. R. Shaver, & L. S. Wrightsman (Eds.), *Measures of personality and social psychological attitudes* (Vol. 1, pp. 61-114). San Diego: Academic Press.

Andrews, F. M., & Withey, S. B. (1976). *Social indicators of well-being.* New York: Plenum.

FALLS EFFICACY SCALE (FES)

AUTHORS: Mary E. Tinetti, Donna Richman, and Lynda Powell
ADDRESS: Mary E. Tinetti, MD
Yale University School of Medicine
333 Cedar Street, PO Box 208025
New Haven, CT 06520-8025

DESCRIPTION: The Falls Efficacy Scale (FES) is an instrument designed to measure fear of falling, operationalized as "low perceived self-efficacy at avoiding falls during essential, nonhazardous activities of daily living" (Tinetti, Richman, & Powell, 1990, p. P239). It was designed by authors interested in the "extent to which fear of falling exerts an independent effect on functional decline in the elderly" (p. P242). FES items inquire about the extent of confidence a respondent has about engaging in 10 selected activities without falling. The scale is not intended for nursing home residents.

PSYCHOMETRIC PROPERTIES: The items for the FES were selected by 10 experts who were asked to identify activities "essential to independent living, that while requiring some position change or walking, would be safe and nonhazardous to most elderly persons" (Tinetti et al., 1990, p. P240). Another group of 10 experts verified the choices providing face validity for the items. Test-retest reliability was estimated (Pearson correlation = 0.71) with a small sample ($N = 18$) of cognitively intact ambulatory community elders who were also asked whether they were afraid of falling and whether fear made them avoid any activities. FES scores were related to fear of falling such that those with low confidence were more likely to say that they avoided activities. FES scores were also associated ($N = 56$) with difficulty getting up after a past fall, trait anxiety, general fear score, and usual walking pace (p. P241). After demonstrating validity and reliability for the instrument with small samples, Tinetti, de Leon, Doucette, and Baker (1994) studied the relationship between fall efficacy and function with a large probability sample of elders ($N = 1,103$) living in the community. Fall-related efficacy was shown to be "a potent independent correlate" of activities of daily living and physical functioning (pp. M143-M144).

PROCEDURE: The respondent rates each of 10 activities on a 10-point scale from *no confidence at all* (0) to *fairly confident/sure* (5) to *completely confident/sure* (10). The scale is designed to be administered in an interview.

SAMPLE ITEMS: "Reaching into cabinets or closets" and "Taking a bath or shower" (Tinetti & Powell, 1993, p. 36).

SCORING: The range of possible total scores, computed as the sum of scores for individual items, is 0 to 100, with low scores corresponding with low self-confidence. The FES may also be scored for the number of items that a respondent rates at 7 or higher, with a range of scores from 0 to 10 (Tinetti et al., 1994, p. M142).

SOURCE: The scale is available from the authors.

REFERENCES

Tinetti, M., Mendes de Leon, C. F., Doucette, J. T., & Baker, D. I. (1994). Fear of falling and fall-related efficacy in relationship to functioning among community-living elders. *Journal of Gerontology: Medical Sciences, 49,* M140-M147.

Tinetti, M., & Powell, L. (1993). Fear of falling and low self-efficacy: A cause of dependence in elderly persons. *Journal of Gerontology, 48,* 35-38.

Tinetti, M. E., Richman, D., & Powell, L. (1990). Falls efficacy as a measure of fear of falling. *Journal of Gerontology: Psychological Sciences, 45,* P239-P243.

FERRANS AND POWERS QUALITY OF LIFE INDEX (FPQLI)

AUTHORS: Carol E. Ferrans and Marjorie J. Powers
ADDRESS: Carol Estwing Ferrans
            Department of Medical-Surgical Nursing
            College of Nursing (M/C 802)
            845 South Damen Avenue, 7th Floor
            University of Illinois at Chicago
            Chicago, IL 60612-7350

DESCRIPTION: The generic version of the Ferrans and Powers Quality of Life Index (FPQLI) is a 68-item instrument designed to measure quality of life in four dimensions: "health and functioning, socioeconomic, psychological/ spiritual, and family" (Ferrans & Powers, 1992, p. 29). It is intended for use by "health care professionals to pinpoint problem areas, examine practices, and plan interventions to improve quality of life" (p. 29). The authors defined quality of life as "a person's sense of well-being that stems from satisfaction or dissatisfaction with the areas of life that are important to him/her" (p. 29). The 34 items of Part I deal with satisfaction. In Part II, 34 items, each paired with an item in Part I, deal with importance. The instrument inquires about satisfaction with an aspect of life as well as the value that it holds for the individual respondent. By adding illness-specific items to the tool's core items, the authors developed versions of the FPQLI for "cardiac, respiratory, cancer, diabetes, arthritis, stroke/head injury, burn, epilepsy, narcolepsy, multiple sclerosis, spinal cord injury/quadriplegic, urostomy, liver transplant, and kidney transplant patients" (p. 37).

PSYCHOMETRIC PROPERTIES: The instrument was originally tested for validity and reliability with samples of graduate students ($n = 88$) and dialysis patients ($n = 37$). Cronbach's alphas were 0.93 and 0.90 respectively (Ferrans & Powers, 1985, p. 20). Test-retest correlations for these samples at 2-week and 1-month intervals respectively (0.87 and 0.81) supported stability of the measure (p. 19). Convergent validity was supported with correlations (0.75 and 0.61) between FPQLI scores and a single-item measure of life satisfaction, assessed with the question "How satisfied are you with your life in general?" Responses could range, on a 6-point scale, from *very satisfied* to *very dissatisfied* (Ferrans & Powers, 1985, p. 19). Ferrans and Powers (1992) later gathered FPQLI data from 349 dialysis patients by mail. Construct validity was studied with factor analysis, analysis of a higher-order factor, and a contrast between scores for known groups (pp. 34-35). Convergent validity for this sample was supported with a correlation between FPQLI and single-item life satisfaction scores (0.77). Alpha coefficients for the total scale (0.93) and subscales (range 0.77 to 0.90) supported internal consistency (p. 36). Further work to validate the psychometric properties of the instrument was conducted with the FPQLI—Cancer Version. Using similar methods, Ferrans (1990) showed internal consistency (alpha = 0.95), concurrent validity (0.80), and higher "quality of life scores for subjects who had less pain, less depression, and were coping better with stress" (p. 15).

PROCEDURE: Subjects respond to a paper-and-pencil instrument. For Part I, responses to each item range on a six-item scale from *very dissatisfied* to *very satisfied.* In Part II, responses range from *very unimportant* to *very important* (Ferrans & Powers, 1985, p. 17).

SAMPLE ITEMS: "How satisfied are you with: The emotional support you get from others?" (Ferrans & Powers, 1984, p. 1) and "How important to you is: The emotional support you get from others?" (Ferrans & Powers, 1984, p. 3).

SCORING: Scores are computed by weighting each "satisfaction" response (Part I) with its paired "importance" response (Part II). Zero is the midpoint of items in Part I, with a range from –2.5 to 2.5. For Part II, the range is between 1 and 6. For each item, the Part I score is multiplied by the score for its Part II counterpart. The overall score is the sum of the weighted scores divided by the number of items answered. "To eliminate negative values, a constant of 15 is added to every score to produce the final score," with the range of possible scores being 0 through 30 (Ferrans & Powers, 1992, p. 31). A computer program to calculate scores is available from the authors.

SOURCE: The copyright for the FPQLI is held by the authors, who must grant permission for its use. In addition to its English version, the FPQLI is available in Japanese, Korean, Mandarin Chinese, Mexican Spanish, Rumanian, and Swedish.

REFERENCES

Ferrans, C. E. (1990). Development of a Quality of Life Index for patients with cancer. *Oncology Nursing Forum, 17*(3), 15-21.

Ferrans, C. E., & Powers, M. J. (1984). *Ferrans and Powers Quality of Life Index.* (Available from the authors at address listed above)

Ferrans, C. E., & Powers, M. J. (1985). Quality of Life Index: Development and psychometric properties. *Advances in Nursing Science, 8*(1), 15-24.

Ferrans, C. E., & Powers, M. J. (1992). Psychometric assessment of the Quality of Life Index. *Research in Nursing and Health, 15,* 29-38.

FROMAJE (FUNCTION, REASONING, ORIENTATION, MEMORY, ARITHMETIC, JUDGMENT, AND EMOTIONAL STATE)

AUTHOR: Leslie S. Libow
ADDRESS: Leslie S. Libow, MD
           Chief of Medical Services
           Jewish Home and Hospital for the Aged
           120 West 106 Street
           New York, NY 10025

DESCRIPTION: The FROMAJE is a rapidly and easily administered test of mental status. It was designed as a guide for "primary care clinicians" with little experience in mental status evaluation. The acronym *FROMAJE* stands for "Function, Reasoning, Orientation, Memory, Arithmetic, Judgment, and Emotional State" (Libow, 1981, p. 87). The technique is not suitable for patients who are aphasic.

PSYCHOMETRIC PROPERTIES: According to Libow (1981), FROMAJE ratings by medical students and lay interviewers had "80% to 90% concordance with the psychiatric diagnoses achieved independently by geropsychiatrists" (p. 87). Rameizl and Pastorello (1984, cited in Doyle, Dunn, Thadani, & Lenihan, 1986) reported figures for internal consistency (0.94) and interrater reliability (0.69) for FROMAJE. Rameizl (1984) used the FROMAJE in conjunction with her measure called CADET (Rameizl, 1983) for routine nursing assessments in a large long-term care setting. *CADET* is an acronym for self-care function: "communication, ambulation, daily living, excretion, transfer."

PROCEDURE: The FROMAJE takes approximately 15 to 20 minutes to administer in an interview. Rapport is established, and the evaluation is introduced generally as the interviewer evaluates the respondent's communication ability. The interviewer says something like "I am going to ask you a series of questions, some of which are simple and some difficult, and the answers to these questions will help me understand how you are functioning" (Libow, 1981, p. 88). The evaluator systematically administers the tests for each of the FROMAJE categories or embeds the items within a longer interview.

SAMPLE ITEMS: "Judgment. 1. At night, if you need some help, how can you obtain it? 2. If you are having trouble with a neighbor, what can you do to improve the situation? 3. If you see smoke in a wastepaper basket, what should you do?" (1 = *Patient made a generally sensible response,* 2 = *Patient demonstrates some poor judgment,* and 3 = *Patient shows extremely poor judgment*) (Libow, 1981, p. 89).

SCORING: Each section of the FROMAJE is rated 1, 2, or 3. The rater matches observations with descriptive statements specified for each item. The range of scores is 7 to 21. Total scores of 7 or 8 indicate no significant abnormal behavior, 9 or 10 suggests mild dementia, 11 or 12 shows moderate dementia or depression, and 13 or higher indicates severe dementia or depression (Libow, 1981, p. 89). An experienced clinician may use the FROMAJE to reach a global impression of mild, moderate, or severe dementia.

SOURCE: The FROMAJE and instructions for administration are printed in Libow (1981). A reprint of the instrument appears in Matteson and McConnell (1988, p. 68).

REFERENCES

Doyle, G. C., Dunn, S. I., Thadani, I., & Lenihan, P. (1986). *Journal of Gerontological Nursing, 12*(9), 19-24.

Libow, L. (1981). A rapidly administered, easily remembered mental status examination: FROMAJE. In L. S. Libow & F. T. Sherman (Eds.), *The core of geriatric medicine* (pp. 85-91). St. Louis: C. V. Mosby.

Matteson, M. A., & McConnell, E. S. (1988). *Gerontological nursing.* Philadelphia: W. B. Saunders.

Rameizl, P. (1983). CADET, a self-care assessment tool. *Geriatric Nursing, 4,* 377-378.

Rameizl, P. (1984). A case for assessment technology in long-term care: The nursing perspective. *Rehabilitation Nursing, 9*(6), 29-31.

FUNCTIONAL ACTIVITIES QUESTIONNAIRE (FAQ)

AUTHOR: Robert I. Pfeffer
ADDRESS: Robert I. Pfeffer, MD
             UCI Study Group, Suite 660
             24411 Health Center Drive
             Laguna Hills, CA 92653-3633

DESCRIPTION: The Functional Activities Questionnaire (FAQ), an index of social function, was designed as a screening tool for use in community studies of normal aging and mild senile dementia. Respondents—informants who are spouses, relatives, or caregivers with at least 3 years of acquaintance and at least a monthly contact—rate the subject on ability to keep records, fill out papers, shop alone, play games of skill, use the stove, prepare a meal, and travel independently; awareness of current events, concentration, and memory are also rated.

PSYCHOMETRIC PROPERTIES: To generate items for the FAQ, the author asked elders participating in a study to validate an instrument that would distinguish between normal aging and mild dementia to rate themselves on their abilities with selected instrumental activities of daily living. Ten functional areas were identified for the FAQ. The instrument was initially tested with a sample of 195 community-dwelling elders. Each participant was examined independently by two neurologists or by a neurologist and a nurse. Data for the FAQ were gathered from informants. Test-retest reliability was estimated for 74 subjects with weighted kappa (0.99). The proportion of agreement between two independent observers rating the same subject ($N = 83$) within 3 months was 0.97 (Pfeffer, 1995, p. 459). FAQ scores were correlated (0.72) with scores on the Instrumental Activities of Daily Living (IADL) Scale (Lawton & Brody, 1969). Residual function was estimated during the neurological examinations ($N = 195$); these estimates were correlated (–0.83) with FAQ scores (Pfeffer, Kurosaki, Harrah, Chance, & Filos, 1982, p. 327). The psychometric properties of the FAQ were reported to compare favorably with those of the IADL scale (Pfeffer et al., 1982, p. 328).

PROCEDURE: The instrument, a paper-and-pencil test, has been used in mail surveys. It could also be used in clinical settings. The person administering the questionnaire may read it to the respondent. Instructions appear on the questionnaire.

SAMPLE ITEM:

Keeps track of current events either in the neighborhood or nationally.

A. Pays no attention to, or doesn't remember outside happenings.
B. Some idea about *major* events (for example, comments on presidential election, major events in the news or major sporting events).
C. Somewhat less attention to, or knowledge of, current events than formerly.

D. As aware of current events as ever was.

E. Never paid much attention to current events, and would find quite difficult to start now.

F. Never paid much attention, but can do as well as anyone now when they try. (Pfeffer, 1980, p. 3)

SCORING: There are four levels of function for each activity item. Weights are assigned to the levels. *Dependent* = 3, *Requires assistance* = 2, *Has difficulty but does by self* = 1, *Normal* = 0, *Never did and would have difficulty now* = 1, and *Never did but could do now* = 0. Total FAQ scores (FAQSUM) are summations of the item scores.

SOURCE: Copies of the original FAQ (Pfeffer, 1980), which is in the public domain, and instructions for scoring the instrument are available from the author. For a later version of the FAQ (since 1984), the author owns a copyright.

REFERENCES

Lawton, M. P., & Brody, E. M. (1969). Assessment of older people: Self-maintaining and instrumental activities of daily living. *Gerontologist, 9,* 179-186.

Pfeffer, R. I. (1980). *Functional Activities Questionnaire.* (Available from the author at address listed above)

Pfeffer, R. I. (1995). A social function measure in the staging and study of dementia. In M. Bergener, J. C. Brocklehurst, & S. I. Finkel (Eds.), *Aging, health, and healing* (pp. 459-474). New York: Springer.

Pfeffer, R. I., Kurosaki, T. T., Harrah, C. H., Chance, J. M., & Filos, S. (1982). Measurement of functional activities in older adults in the community. *Journal of Gerontology, 3,* 323-329.

FUNCTIONAL ASSESSMENT STAGING (FAST)

AUTHOR: Barry Reisberg

ADDRESS: Barry Reisberg, MD
            Aging and Dementia Research Center
            New York University Medical Center
            550 First Avenue
            New York, NY 10016

DESCRIPTION: The Functional Assessment Staging (FAST) is a 16-item hierarchical scale for assessing a person's ability to perform basic activities of daily life. Its items represent an ordinal sequence of functional loss characteristic of dementia. The FAST is one of the elements of the Global Deterioration Scale staging system developed by Reisberg and his colleagues (see entry in this book); it can also be used as an independent clinical rating. Scores on the FAST range between Stage 1 (normal) and Stage 7 (severe dementia). Stages 6 and 7 have subdivisions. The FAST is especially "useful for the detailed staging and substaging of severe and very severe Alzheimer's disease" (Reisberg et al., 1993, p. S53).

PSYCHOMETRIC PROPERTIES: Convergent validity of the FAST has been supported ($N = 566$) by a correlation (0.83) between FAST and Mini-Mental State Examination (MMSE; see entry in this book) scores (Sclan & Reisberg, 1992, p. 20). The most severely impaired, however, had scores of 0 on the MMSE. Validity for the FAST at these lower levels needed to be substantiated. On the basis of the theory that patterns of loss in Alzheimer's disease were similar to those of acquisition of cognitive ability in normal development, Reisberg and his colleagues correlated FAST scores, for persons at FAST levels of 6 and 7 ($N = 38$), with their scores on a modified scale usually used to trace early development. The developmental scores correlated with the FAST at 0.79 ($p < 0.001$) (Reisberg, Sclan, Franssen, Kluger, & Ferris, 1994, p. S196). Reliability of the FAST has been demonstrated in several small studies. When two clinical fellows simultaneously rated 16 elderly patients with various levels of dementia and their caregivers (Sclan & Reisberg, 1992), intraclass correlation coefficients (ICCs) were 0.88 for rater consistency and 0.87 for rater agreement. An ICC of 0.96 was achieved when five attending psychiatrists simultaneously rated 20 long-term care patients. The ICC was 0.76, however, when simultaneous ratings were performed ($N = 20$) by three research assistants, a nurse, a psychologist, and a graduate student (Reisberg, 1988).

PROCEDURE: The interviewer compares observed behaviors and/or information supplied by caregivers who have knowledge of the patient with specific descriptions in annotated guidelines. "The highest consecutive level of disability" is recorded by the interviewer (Reisberg et al., 1994, p. S195).

SAMPLE ITEMS:

Stage 5: "Deficient performance in choosing proper attire, and assistance is required for independent community functioning" (Sclan & Reisberg, 1992, p. 58).

Stage 6a: "Requires actual physical assistance in putting on clothing properly" (Sclan & Reisberg, 1992, p. 58).

SCORING: "The FAST stage is the highest ordinally enumerated score" (Sclan & Reisberg, 1992, p. 59). Detailed annotated guidelines for scoring are printed in Reisberg (1988).

SOURCE: The instrument is available from the author, who holds its copyright. It has been reprinted in Reisberg (1988) and Sclan and Reisberg (1992).

REFERENCES

Reisberg, B. (1988). Functional Assessment Staging (FAST). *Psychopharmacology Bulletin, 24,* 653-659.

Reisberg, B., Sclan, S. G., Franssen, E., deLeon, M. J., Kluger, A., Torossian, C., Shulman, E., Steinberg, G., Monteiro, I., McRae, T., Boksay, I., Mackell, J., & Ferris, S. H. (1993). Clinical stages of normal aging and Alzheimer's disease: The GDS staging system. *Neuroscience Research Communications, 13*(Suppl. 1), S51-S54.

Reisberg, B., Sclan, S. G., Franssen, E., Kluger, A., & Ferris, S. (1994). Dementia staging in chronic care populations. *Alzheimer Disease and Associated Disorders, 8*(Suppl. 1), S188-S205.

Sclan, S. G., & Reisberg, B. (1992). Functional Assessment Staging (FAST) in Alzheimer's disease: Reliability, validity, and ordinality. *International Psychogeriatrics, 4*(Suppl. 1), 55-69.

FUNCTIONAL REACH

AUTHORS: Pamela W. Duncan, Debra K. Weiner, Stephanie Studenski, and Julie Chandler

ADDRESS: Dr. Pamela W. Duncan
            Graduate Program in Physical Therapy
            P.O. Box 3965
            Duke University Medical Center
            Durham, NC 27710

DESCRIPTION: Functional reach is a dynamic, interval-level measure of balance, or postural control. Duncan, Weiner, Chandler, and Studenski (1990) defined functional reach as "the maximal distance one can reach forward beyond arm's length while maintaining a fixed base of support in the standing position" (p. M192). The technique, which is inexpensive, is simple to perform, and yields a precise score representing balance, may be used to detect balance problems that put individuals at risk for falls and to assess changes in balance following interventions and over time.

PSYCHOMETRIC PROPERTIES: Male and female hospital employees, physical therapy students, and community-dwelling elderly ($N = 128$) were subjects in the initial trials. Their ages ranged between 20 and 87; 34 persons in the sample were over 70. Criterion validity was established with strong associations between functional reach and COPE (center of pressure excursion). COPE is defined as the difference between the location of the center of pressure during relaxed standing and maximum forward reach. Concurrent validity was demonstrated ($N = 45$) with strong correlations between functional reach and other measures of physical performance, such as walking speed, instrumental activities of daily living, one-foot standing, and tandem walking in a community-dwelling sample aged 66 to 104 (Weiner, Duncan, Chandler, & Studenski, 1992). Duncan, Studenski, Chandler, and Prescott (1992) demonstrated that the measure predicted recurrent falls among elderly community-dwelling men ($N = 215$) aged 70 and over who were attending ambulatory care clinics. On test-retest, functional reach was highly reproducible, with intraclass correlation coefficients (ICC) of 0.92 ($N = 14$; Duncan et al., 1990, p. M195) and 0.89 ($N = 13$; Weiner et al., 1992, p. 206). Interrater reliability was demonstrated with ICC for 17 interobserver measurements at 0.98. Information about the instrument's responsiveness to change is not yet available.

PROCEDURE: The technique comprises the following steps:

1. Mount a 48-inch "yardstick," with capability of adjustment for height, on a wall.
2. Use a leveling device to ensure that the yardstick is parallel with the floor.
3. Adjust yardstick so that it is level with the subject's shoulder (acromion).
4. Be prepared to guard the subject throughout the procedure.

5. Ask subject to (a) stand comfortably, (b) make a fist, and (c) raise arm (right or left, depending on right- or left-handedness) parallel with the yardstick. This is Position #1.
6. Record point on yardstick parallel to the third knuckle (metacarpal).
7. Ask subject to reach as far forward as possible, with his or her fist at the level of the ruler, without losing balance, taking a step, or touching the wall (Position #2).
8. Record point on yardstick parallel to the third metacarpal.

If the subject touches the wall or takes a step, a trial is invalid. The subject repeats the procedure five times. The score is calculated from data gathered during the last three trials. The investigator can substitute large sheets of graph paper with 1-inch squares secured to a wall. Use a level to ensure that lines are parallel to the floor. Mark the specific line on the paper at the level of the acromion. When the subject reaches to establish Position #2, he or she reaches with reference to the marked line.

SCORING: The score for functional reach is the mean difference between Position #1 and Position #2. Subtract the score for Position #1 from the score for Position #2 for each trial. Add the three resulting numbers together, and divide that sum by 3.

SOURCE: The procedure is specified in the article describing the test (Duncan et al., 1990).

REFERENCES

Duncan, P. W., Studenski, S., Chandler, J., & Prescott, B. (1992). Functional reach: Predictive validity in a sample of elderly male veterans. *Journal of Gerontology: Medical Sciences, 47,* M93-M98.
Duncan, P. W., Weiner, D. K., Chandler, J., & Studenski, S. (1990). Functional reach: A new clinical balance measure. *Journal of Gerontology: Medical Sciences, 45,* M192-M197.
Weiner, D. K., Duncan, P. W., Chandler, J., & Studenski, S. A. (1992). Functional reach: A marker of physical frailty. *Journal of the American Geriatrics Society, 40,* 203-207.

GENERAL WELL-BEING SCHEDULE (GWB)

AUTHOR: Harold J. Dupuy
ADDRESS: U.S. Department of Health and Human Services
            Public Health Services
            Centers for Disease Control and Prevention
            National Center for Health Statistics
            6525 Belcrest Road
            Hyattsville, MD 20782

DESCRIPTION: The General Well-Being Schedule (GWB) is a "self report instrument designed to assess selected aspects of self-representations of subjective well-being and distress" (Dupuy, 1977, p. iii). The schedule was developed by Dupuy in 1970 at the National Center for Health Statistics (NCHS). It has been used with many thousands of subjects in diverse populations. The GWB is a 33-item instrument with six subscales to measure "health worry, energy level, satisfying interesting life, depressed-cheerful mood, emotional behavioral control, and relaxed versus tense-anxious" (Fazio, 1977, p. 4).

PSYCHOMETRIC PROPERTIES: In 1977, the NCHS published the instrument in a report by Fazio about GWB data gathered from 195 college students. GWB scores and scores from other mental health scales gathered concurrently were compared with interviewers' ratings of depression. The GWB distinguished between depressed and nondepressed students and was better than other measures in its strength of relationship with interviewer ratings for depression (Fazio, 1977, p. 12). Himmelfarb and Murrell (1983) conducted a study to assess the validity and reliability of five mental health scales that they used with older persons. They found better discrimination—between community-dwelling and psychiatric patient samples—for the GWB than for the other scales they evaluated. Alpha coefficients showed high internal validity for the GWB with both community (0.88) and psychiatric patient (0.91) samples. Costa et al. (1987) analyzed longitudinal data gathered at a 9-year interval from a large representative national sample (National Health and Nutrition Examination Survey) using 10 items of the GWB. Results showed that subjective well-being had not declined with age, providing "compelling evidence for the stability of levels of well-being in adulthood" (p. 54). Nickel, Brown, and Smith (1990) measured anxiety and depression in heart disease survivors using two questions from the GWB that had been shown to have correlated well with total GWB scores (Fazio, 1977, p. 23).

PROCEDURE: The GWB is a paper-and-pencil test with clear instructions printed on the test form. For the first 18 items, the subject is directed to respond for the period "during the past month."

SAMPLE ITEM:

Have you been under or felt you were under any strain, stress, or pressure? (DURING THE PAST MONTH).

1. Yes—almost more than I could bear or stand
2. Yes—quite a bit of pressure
3. Yes—some—more than usual
4. Yes—some—but about usual
5. Yes—a little
6. Not at all (Fazio, 1977, p. 1)

SCORING: The first 14 items have six possible response options; 4 items have bar scale responses that may range from 0 to 10. To code the responses for analysis, investigators follow guidelines on the GWB Case Record Summary Sheet. The range of scores for the 18 items is 14 to 124, with high scores indicating greater well-being. There are 15 additional items that focus on criterion variables in areas such as seeking professional help, history of "nervous breakdown," fear of "nervous breakdown," and social-emotional support.

SOURCE: The user will need the GWB Case Record Summary Sheet as well as the GWB schedule itself. Both are reproduced in the appendix to Fazio (1977), a publication available from the NCHS.

REFERENCES

Costa, P. T., Zonderman, A. B., McCrae, R. R., Cornoni-Huntley, J., Locke, B. Z., & Barbano, H. E. (1987). Longitudinal analyses of psychological well-being in a national sample. *Journal of Gerontology, 42,* 50-55.

Dupuy, H. J. (1977). Foreword. In A. F. Fazio, *A concurrent validation study of the NCHS General Well-Being Schedule* (pp. iii-iv, DHEW Pub. No. HRA-78-1347, Vital and Health Statistics, Series 2, No. 73). Hyattsville, MD: National Center for Health Statistics.

Fazio, A. F. (1977). *A concurrent validation study of the NCHI General Well-Being Schedule* (DHEW Pub. No. HRA-78-1347, Vital and Health Statistics, Series 2, No. 73). Hyattsville, MD: National Center for Health Statistics.

Himmelfarb, S., & Murrell, S. A. (1983). Reliability and validity of five mental health scales in older persons. *Journal of Gerontology, 38,* 333-339.

Nickel, J. T., Brown, K. J., & Smith, B. A. (1990). Depression and anxiety among chronically ill heart patients: Age differences in risk and predictors. *Research in Nursing and Health, 13,* 87-97.

GERIATRIC DEPRESSION SCALE (GDS)

AUTHORS: Jerome A. Yesavage, Thomas L. Brink, Terence L. Rose, Owen Lum, Virginia Huang, Michael Adey, and Von Otto Leirer

ADDRESS: Thomas L. Brink, PhD, MBA
1103 North Church Street
Redlands, CA 92374

DESCRIPTION: The Geriatric Depression Scale (GDS) is a tool for screening depression in the elderly. It has a simple yes-no response format that is easy to complete. References to somatic complaints, sleep disturbances, and sexual function were not included in the GDS because changes in these phenomena are known to be associated with normal aging. The tool, which is "not a substitute for observer-rated scales or in depth diagnostic interviews" (Yesavage et al., 1983, p. 48) has a 30-item long form and a 15-item short form (Sheikh & Yesavage, 1986).

PSYCHOMETRIC PROPERTIES: In the initial phases of instrument development, experts selected 100 items that could discriminate between depressed and nondepressed elders. Thirty of the 100, those demonstrating highest correlations with total scores, were selected for the instrument. Validity was supported when GDS scores differentiated between "normal," "mildly depressed," and "severely depressed" groups of elders ($N = 100$) identified clinically with criteria symptoms for a major affective disorder (Yesavage et al., 1983, p. 42). Correlations between GDS scores and scores on two other measures of depression showed convergent validity. Correlations for test-retest scores ($N = 20$) at a 1-week interval (0.85), and split-half reliability coefficients (0.94) demonstrated that the measure was reliable

(Yesavage et al., 1983). Internal consistency was shown by an alpha coefficient of 0.94.

PROCEDURE: The GDS may be administered in an interview or completed by the subject as a self-report. With frail elders, an oral format is preferred. The examiner may have to repeat the items to get a response that is clearly a "yes" or a "no."

SAMPLE ITEMS: "Do you feel full of energy?" and "Do you prefer to avoid social gatherings?" (Yesavage et al., 1983, p. 41).

SCORING: For the 30-item form, 10 items indicate depression when they are answered "no." The other 20 items indicate depression when they are answered "yes." Norms for the long form are: 0 to 10 = normal; 11 to 20 = mild depression; and 21 to 30 = moderate or severe depression. See Sheikh and Yesavage (1986) for short-form norms.

SOURCE: The long form of the scale is reprinted in Yesavage et al. (1983); the short form appears in Sheikh and Yesavage (1986).

REFERENCES

Sheikh, J. I., & Yesavage, J. A. (1986). Geriatric Depression Scale (GDS): Recent findings and development of a shorter version. *Clinical Gerontologist, 5,* 165-173.

Yesavage, J. A., Brink, T. L., Rose, T. L., Lum, O., Huang, V., Adey, M., & Leirer, V. O. (1983). Development and validation of a geriatric depression screening scale: A preliminary report. *Journal of Psychiatric Research, 17,* 37-49.

GERIATRIC HOPELESSNESS SCALE (GERIHS)

AUTHOR: P. S. Fry
ADDRESS: Professor P. S. Fry
            Department of Educational Psychology
            University of Calgary
            Calgary, Alberta T2N 1N4, Canada

DESCRIPTION: The Geriatric Hopelessness Scale (GERIHS) is an instrument for "assessment of pessimism and cognitions of hopelessness in elderly clients" (Fry, 1986, p. 193). The author defined hopelessness as "negative expectancies toward oneself, the world, and the future" (p. 195). The scale has 30 items that "refer to the affective, motivational and cognitive components of hopelessness in the subject" (p. 195).

PSYCHOMETRIC PROPERTIES: To derive GERIHS items, the author analyzed the content of interviews with 60 Canadian elders who resided in the community (Fry, 1984, p. 324). A list of 52 statements reflecting current or future pessimism was compiled and submitted to factor analysis. Four themes were identified:

1. A sense of hopelessness about recovering lost physical and cognitive abilities
2. A sense of hopelessness about recovering lost personal and interpersonal worth
3. A sense of hopelessness about recovering spiritual faith and receiving spiritual grace
4. A sense of hopelessness about receiving nurturance and recovering respect and remembrance (p. 324)

Items with substantial factor loadings were selected for subsequent testing with a different sample of retired white Canadians ($N = 78$) aged 60 to 80 years. In addition to the GERIHS, the subjects responded to the Geriatric Depression Scale (see entry in this book) and the Tennessee Self-Concept Scale (Fitts, 1965) and were rated for behavioral symptoms of depression by family members or a social worker. Internal consistency for the GERIHS was estimated with Cronbach's alpha (0.69; p. 327). Item-to-total score correlations ranged between 0.31 and 0.71, with an average correlation of 0.57. Fry (1984) correlated GERIHS scores with GDS scores (0.49) and with the ratings of behavioral depression (0.55). When the sample was divided by high and low hopelessness scores, those with high scores had higher depression scores and lower self-concept scores.

PROCEDURE: The scale can be administered in either oral or written formats. There are 15 items keyed to be answered "true" for hopelessness, interspersed with 15 items keyed for "false." The items are written at a junior high school reading level.

SAMPLE ITEMS: "All I can see ahead of me is more grief and sadness"; "Even as an elderly person, I can be useful and helpful to others"; "I believe that my family and friends will miss me after I'm gone"; and "I've never had much luck in the past, and there's no reason to think I will, now that I'm old and tired" (Fry, 1984, p. 326).

SCORING: The range of scores is 0 to 30, with higher scores indicating greater hopelessness. Cutoff scores were suggested by Fry (1986). Scores between 0 and 10 show low hopelessness, scores between 11 and 19 indicate moderate levels and a need for help and moral support, and scores between 20 and 30 indicate high levels of hopelessness with clinical despair and the need for prompt professional help (Fry, 1986, p. 197).

SOURCE: Copies of the items on the GERIHS appear in Fry (1984, 1986).

REFERENCES

Fitts, W. H. (1965). *Manual for the Tennessee Self Concept Scale.* Los Angeles: Western Psychological Services.

Fry, P. S. (1984). The development of a geriatric scale of hopelessness: Implications for counseling and intervention with depressed elderly. *Journal of Clinical Psychology, 31,* 322-331.

Fry, P. S. (1986). Assessment of pessimism and despair: A geriatric scale of hopelessness. *Clinical Gerontologist, 5,* 193-201.

GLASGOW COMA SCALE (GCS)

AUTHORS: Graham Teasdale and Bryan Jennett
ADDRESS: Professor Graham Teasdale
             Department of Neurosurgery
             University of Glasgow
             Institute of Neurological Sciences
             The Southern General Hospital
             Glasgow G51 4TF, Scotland

DESCRIPTION: The Glasgow Coma Scale (GCS) was designed to assess the depth and duration of impaired consciousness and coma (Teasdale & Jennett, 1974). It is a method for making standardized observations for eye opening, verbal behavior, and motor responsiveness. The GCS facilitates consistent observations and accurate communication about levels of consciousness. It is useful for systematically defining the duration of a prolonged coma (p. 81). Procedures are simple and practical, but they require that observers study guidelines and practice assessments. The GCS has been used in assessment of patients with end-stage Alzheimer's disease (Benesch, McDaniel, Cox, & Hamill, 1993).

PSYCHOMETRIC PROPERTIES: The scale evolved from clinical work with head injury patients. Reliability of the instrument was estimated by Stanczak et al. (1984) in three ways ($N = 101$): internal consistency (0.86), interrater reliability (0.95), and test-retest (0.85) reliability (p. 957). Validity of the GCS was demonstrated when depths of comas measured with the GCS were related, in rank order, to patient outcomes (Jennett, Teasdale, & Knill-Jones, 1975, p. 235). There have been some reports that question the reliability and validity of GCS assessments (Segatore & Way, 1992). Improving the properties seems to rest with training. Teasdale, Knill-Jones, and Van Der Sande (1978) showed that experience in the use of the scale reduced observer variability.

PROCEDURE: Using detailed instructions, the observer rates (a) eye opening, (b) verbal response, and (c) motor response. The authors developed special graphic sheets for charting GCS observations. They appear in Teasdale (1975) and Teasdale, Galbraith, and Clarke (1975). GCS guidelines are published in Jones (1979).

SAMPLE ITEM: Eye Opening: The observer rates opening of eyes as "spontaneous," only in response "to speech," only in response "to pain," or "none" (Teasdale & Jennett, 1974, p. 84).

SCORING: Jones (1979) reported a coding scheme in which the range of total scores is between 3 and 14. For assessment of eye opening, the range of scores is from 4 to 1, and for assessment of verbal response and motor responses, scores range from 5 to 1.

SOURCE: Copyright for the GCS is held between Drs. Teasdale and Jennett and the *Lancet.*

REFERENCES

Benesch, C. G., McDaniel, K. D., Cox, C., & Hamill, R. W. (1993). End-stage Alzheimer's disease: Glasgow Coma Scale and the neurologic examination. *Archives of Neurology, 50,* 1309-1315.

Jennett, B., Teasdale, G. M., & Knill-Jones, R. P. (1975). Predicting outcome after head injury. *Journal of the Royal College of Physicians of London, 9,* 231-237.

Jones, C. (1979). Glasgow Coma Scale. *American Journal of Nursing, 79,* 1551-1553.

Segatore, M., & Way, C. (1992). The Glasgow Coma Scale: Time for change. *Heart and Lung, 21,* 548-557.

Stanczak, D. E., White, J. G., Gouview, W. D., Moehle, K. A., Daniel, M., Novack, T., & Long, C. J. (1984). Assessment of level of consciousness following severe neurological insult: A comparison of the psychometric qualities of the Glasgow Coma Scale and the Comprehensive Level of Consciousness Scale. *Journal of Neurosurgery, 60,* 955-960.

Teasdale, G. (1975, June 12). Acute impairment of brain function 1: Assessing "conscious level." *Nursing Times,* pp. 914-917.

Teasdale, G., Galbraith, S., & Clarke, K. (1975, June 19). Acute impairment of brain function 2: Observation record chart. *Nursing Times,* pp. 972-973.

Teasdale, G., & Jennett, B. (1974). Assessment of coma and impaired consciousness: A practical scale. *Lancet, 2*(7872), 81-84.

Teasdale, G., Knill-Jones, R., & Van Der Sande, J. (1978). Observer variability in assessing impaired consciousness and coma. *Journal of Neurology, Neurosurgery, and Psychiatry, 41,* 603-610.

GLOBAL DETERIORATION SCALE (GLDS)

AUTHORS: Barry Reisberg, Steven H. Ferris, Mony J. deLeon, and Thomas Crook

ADDRESS: Barry Reisberg, MD, Clinical Director
Aging and Dementia Research Center
New York University Medical Center
550 Fifth Avenue
New York, NY 10016

DESCRIPTION: The Global Deterioration Scale (GLDS) is a 7-point rating instrument used for staging the magnitude of "cognitive and functional capacity in normal aging, age-associated memory impairment, and primary degenerative dementia" (Reisberg, Ferris, deLeon, & Crook, 1988, p. 661). The GLDS is part of a staging system for clinical assessment of persons with Alzheimer's disease (AD) that also includes Functional Assessment Staging and the Brief Cognitive Rating Scale (see entries in this book). Each of the seven stages in the GLDS is identified by clinical characteristics. The descriptions of the scale delineate the progression of AD from the earliest to the most severe stages (Reisberg, Ferris, deLeon, & Crook, 1982, p. 1139). Ehrlich and White (1991) developed a program for caregivers of persons with AD using a GLDS-based model to guide planning for respite services.

PSYCHOMETRIC PROPERTIES: During the initial 5 years of their work, the authors conducted interviews with thousands of patients. They described the stages of AD "on the basis of systematic phenomenologic observations" (Reisberg, Sclan, Franssen, Kluger, & Ferris, 1994, p. S189). Later, these descriptions became the detailed clinical criteria for the GLDS. Reanalyses of the phrases used in the GLDS descriptions supported content validity for the scale (p. S190). Validity was also demonstrated ($N = 154$) with correlations between GLDS ratings and scores on Folstein's Mini-Mental State Examination (see entry in this book; 0.89, $p < 0.001$) and between the GLDS and a composite psychometric measure for a group ($N = 251$) of aged and AD subjects (0.86, $p < 0.001$). Test-retest reliability at 1 to 4 weeks (0.82 to 0.92) and interrater reliability for staging of dementia (0.92 to 0.97) were estimated in four studies (pp. S190-S191).

PROCEDURE: Data used to rate the GLDS are gathered in a clinician's interview.

SAMPLE ITEM:

> Stage 4, Moderate Cognitive Decline: Clear-cut deficit on careful clinical interview. Deficit manifest in following areas: (a) decreased knowledge of current and recent events; (b) may exhibit some deficit in memory of one's personal history; (c) concentration deficit elicited on serial subtractions; (d) decreased ability to travel, handle finances, etc. Frequently no deficit in following areas: (a) orientation to time and person; (b) recognition of familiar persons and faces; (c) ability to travel to familiar locations. Inability to perform complex tasks. Denial is dominant defense mechanism. Flattening of affect and withdrawal from challenging situations occur. (Reisberg et al., 1988, p. 661)

SCORING: Using the clinical descriptions of the scale as the rating criteria, the clinician assigns one of seven stages for the subject's level of cognitive functioning.

SOURCE: The scale is copyrighted by Dr. Reisberg. Copies of the instrument are reprinted in Reisberg et al. (1982, 1988).

REFERENCES

Ehrlich, P., & White, J. (1991). TOPS: A consumer approach to Alzheimer's respite programs. *Gerontologist, 31,* 686-691.

Reisberg, B., Ferris, S. H., deLeon, M. J., & Crook, T. (1982). The Global Deterioration Scale for assessment of primary degenerative dementia. *American Journal of Psychiatry, 139,* 1136-1139.

Reisberg, B., Ferris, S. H., deLeon, M. J., & Crook, T. (1988). *Psychopharmacological Bulletin, 24,* 661-663.

Reisberg, B., Sclan, S. G., Franssen, E., Kluger, A., & Ferris, S. (1994). Dementia staging in chronic care populations. *Alzheimer Disease and Associated Disorders, 8*(Suppl. 1), S188-S205.

GOTTSCHALK HOPE SCALE (GHS)

AUTHOR: Louis A. Gottschalk
ADDRESS: Louis A. Gottschalk, MD, PhD
            Professor of Psychiatry and Social Science
            Department of Psychiatry and Human Behavior
            College of Medicine
            University of California Irvine
            Irvine, CA 92717

DESCRIPTION: The Gottschalk Hope Scale (GHS) is a method for analyzing the magnitude of hopefulness projected in verbal behaviors. Samples of speech are analyzed for seven content categories related to hope and hopelessness. When scores for the categories are averaged, the resulting hope score provides an approximation of a measure for a psychological trait (Gottschalk, 1974, p. 782). The GHS is part of a larger content analysis method (Gottschalk, 1995; Gottschalk & Gleser, 1969; Gottschalk, Winget, & Gleser, 1969) proposed to measure the magnitude of many different psychological states and traits. In addition to the scale for hope, there are scales for anxiety, hostility, social alienation/personal disorganization, cognitive and intellectual impairment, and depression (Gottschalk & Bechtel, 1993).

PSYCHOMETRIC PROPERTIES: Technicians who scored early validation samples were trained until they reached interscorer agreement of 85% or higher (Gottschalk, 1974, p. 780). Scales may now be analyzed reliably with a computer program developed by the author (Gottschalk, 1995; Gottschalk & Bechtel, 1993). The validity of the scale has been supported in many different ways. It has face validity based on the author's definition of hope: "A measure of optimism that a favorable outcome is likely to occur, not only in one's personal earthly activities but also in cosmic phenomena and even spiritual or imaginary events" (Gottschalk, 1974, p. 779). Hope scores for mental health patients attending a crisis intervention clinic (–0.45) were significantly lower than scores for a normative adult group (0.73). A low but statistically significant correlation was found between pre-treatment Hope scores and improvement in psychiatric patients (p. 783). Hope scores of schizophrenic patients were significantly correlated with their scores on other psychiatric ratings. Preradiation hope scores of cancer patients correlated significantly with their survival. Patients who followed through with treatment recommendations had higher scores than those who did not. Recently, Gottschalk, Fronczek, and Buchsbaum (1993) reported findings from a study of 10 young men that "provide an initial glimpse into the cerebral neurobiology of the psychological dimensions of states of hopefulness and hopelessness" (p. 279). Positive and negative hope scores were correlated with localized cerebral metabolic rates seen with positron emission tomography scanning. The correlations for hopelessness were located in different areas of the brain than the correlations involving hopefulness (p. 277).

PROCEDURE: In original studies to validate the GHS, speech samples were free associations, with choice of content as free from influence by the interviewer as possible. The authors used standardized instructions, such as "This is a study of speaking and conversational habits. I would like you to speak into the microphone of this tape recorder for five minutes about any interesting or dramatic personal life experiences you have ever had" (Gottschalk, 1974, p. 779). These instructions were ambiguous enough to create a projective test "to which the speaker reacts in terms of his preferred response tendencies, both superficial and deep" (p. 780). Audiotapes were transcribed and analyzed with the scale, using the grammatical clause as the smallest unit for analysis.

SAMPLE ITEM: "References to self or others getting or receiving help, advice, support, sustenance, confidence, esteem (a) from others; (b) from self" (Gottschalk et al., 1993, p. 274).

SCORING: Original scoring instructions are available in a manual (Gottschalk et al., 1969). Computer-programmed scoring is discussed in publications by Gottschalk (1995) and Gottschalk and Bechtel (1993).

SOURCE: The GHS is printed in Gottschalk (1974), Gottschalk and Bechtel (1993), and Gottschalk (1995). Information about the computer program to score the Hope Scale and the other Gottschalk scales is available in Gottschalk (1995) and in copyrighted material available from Mind Garden (Gottschalk & Bechtel, 1993).

REFERENCES

Gottschalk, L. A. (1974). A hope scale applicable to verbal samples. *Archives of General Psychiatry, 30,* 779-785.

Gottschalk, L. A. (1995). *Content analysis and verbal behavior.* Hillsdale, NJ: Lawrence Erlbaum.

Gottschalk, L. A., & Bechtel, R. (1993). *Computerized content analysis of natural language for verbal texts.* (Available from Mind Garden, 3803 East Bayshore Road, Palo Alto, CA 94303, telephone (415) 691-9194)

Gottschalk, L. A., Fronczek, J., & Buchsbaum, M. S. (1993). The cerebral neurobiology of hope and hopelessness. *Psychiatry, 56,* 270-281.

Gottschalk, L. A., & Gleser, G. C. (1969). *The measurement of psychological states from the content analysis of verbal behavior.* Berkeley: University of California Press.

Gottschalk, L. A., Winget, C. N., & Gleser, G. C. (1969). *Manual of instructions for use of the Gottschalk-Gleser Content Analysis Scales: Anxiety, Hostility, Social Alienation-Personal Disorganization.* Los Angeles: University of California Press.

HAMILTON ANXIETY RATING SCALE (HARS)

AUTHOR: Max Hamilton

DESCRIPTION: The Hamilton Anxiety Rating Scale (HARS) is a 14-item observer-rated instrument designed to quantify symptoms of anxiety. It was "intended for use with patients already diagnosed as suffering from neurotic anxiety states, not for assessing anxiety in patients suffering from other disorders" (Hamilton, 1959, p. 50). The 14 items are "defined by a series of brief statements headed by the name of the variable" (p. 50). The statements, 89 in all, are symptoms reflecting both psychic and somatic aspects of anxiety. The variable headings are "Anxious Mood, Tension, Fears, Insomnia, Intellectual, Depressed Mood, Somatic (Muscular), Somatic (Sensory), Cardiovascular Symptoms, Gastrointestinal Symptoms, Genitourinary Symptoms, Autonomic Symptoms, and Behavior in Interview" (p. 50). The instrument was used in the 1970s in the Early Clinical Drug Evaluation Unit Studies (Guy, 1976). In 1979, Kochansky noted that none of the observer rating scales focusing exclusively on symptoms of anxiety was designed specifically for the elderly. However, the HARS, he said, "may have some utility in geriatric psychopharmacology" (p. 138). According to Sheikh (1992), the HARS is the most popular observer-rated scale to measure anxiety and "the standard in the field as a measure of change in clinical situations and in pharmacological research" (p. 418). The scale has been used widely in psychopharmacological studies including several with older adults (Covington, 1975; Kirven & Montero, 1973; Nair et al., 1993).

PSYCHOMETRIC PROPERTIES: The author assembled a list of symptoms "to cover the condition adequately" (Hamilton, 1959, p. 50). The symptoms were grouped together "according to their nature or where clinical experiences indicated that they were associated" (p. 50). Initially, 12 groupings, plus an item for "Behavior in the Interview," were chosen "for practical purposes" (p. 50). Later, the single "Somatic" category was divided to become two variables: "Somatic (Muscular)" and "Somatic (Sensory)." The author conducted several pilot studies as he refined the instrument. Reliability was estimated with ratings by three psychiatrists on a group of patients ($N = 35$) who were seen by pairs of raters simultaneously (p. 51). One psychiatrist conducted the interview, and the other observed and asked questions if more information was needed. Ratings were made independently and were judged reliable; a weighted mean correlation was 0.89 (p. 51). The author investigated whether raters had been biased; that is, consistent in having given higher or lower ratings. Results showed "very little bias" (p. 51). The correlations between variables could be "factorized into a general factor of anxiety and a bipolar factor contrasting psychic with somatic symptoms; or into two orthogonal group factors of 'psychic' and 'somatic' anxiety" (p. 53).

PROCEDURE: The clinician conducts an interview and rates each item on a 5-point scale. The author pointed out that the highest rating, "very severe, grossly disabling," will rarely be used for outpatients (Hamilton, 1959, p. 50).

SAMPLE ITEM: "Anxious Mood. Worries, anticipation of the worst, fearful anticipation, irritability" (Guy, 1976, p. 194).

SCORING: Each of the 14 items is rated on a 5-point scale:

0 = *not present*, 1 = *mild*, 2 = *moderate*, 3 = *severe,* and 4 = *very severe.*
Range of total scores is from 0 to 56.

SOURCE: The scale appears in Hamilton (1959) and is reprinted in Guy (1976).

REFERENCES

Covington, J. S. (1975). Alleviating agitation, apprehension, and related symptoms in geriatric patients: A double-blind comparison of phenothiazine and a benzodiazepine. *Southern Medical Journal, 68,* 719-724.

Guy, W. (1976). *Early Clinical Drug Evaluation Unit assessment manual for psychopharmacology* (Rev. ed., DHEW Pub. No. ADM 76-338). Washington, DC: U.S. Department of Health, Education and Welfare.

Hamilton, M. (1959). The assessment of anxiety states by rating. *British Journal of Medical Psychology, 32,* 50-55.

Kirven, L. E., & Montero, E. F. (1973). Comparison of thioridazine and diazepam in the control of nonpsychotic symptoms associated with senility: Double-blind study. *Journal of the American Geriatrics Society, 21,* 546-551.

Kochansky, G. E. (1979). Psychiatric rating scales for assessing psychopathology in the elderly: A critical review. In A. Raskin & L. Jarvik (Eds.), *Psychiatric symptoms and cognitive loss in the elderly* (pp. 125-156). Washington, DC: Hemisphere.

Nair, N. P., Amin, M., Schwartz, G., Dastoor, D., Thavunday, J. X., Mirmiran, J., MacDonald, C., & Phillips, R. (1993). A comparison of the cardiac safety and therapeutic efficacy of trimipramine versus doxepin in geriatric depressed patients. *Journal of the American Geriatrics Society, 41,* 863-867.

Sheikh, J. I. (1992). Anxiety and its disorders in old age. In J. E. Birren, R. B. Sloane, G. D. Cohen, N. R. Hooyman, B. D. Lebowitz, M. Wykle, & D. E. Deutchman (Eds.), *Handbook of mental health and aging* (2nd ed., pp. 409-432). San Diego: Academic Press.

HAYCOX DEMENTIA BEHAVIOR SCALE (HDBS)

AUTHOR: James A. Haycox
ADDRESS: James A. Haycox, MD
           The Burke Rehabilitation Center
           785 Mamaroneck Avenue
           White Plains, NY 10605

DESCRIPTION: The Haycox Dementia Behavior Scale (HDBS) is an instrument designed to fill the need for a "simple behavioral rating scale for evaluating demented patients" (Haycox, 1984, p. 23). The scale is easy to administer and allows an observer to assess eight categories of potential behavior deficits: "language-conversation, social interaction, attention-awareness, spatial orientation, motor coordination, bowel and bladder, eating and nutrition, and dress and grooming" (Haycox, 1984, p. 24). Items in each category describe behaviors arranged in order of increasing severity. Rosswurm (1989) used scores on the scale as indicators of the presence and degree of dementia. Other nurses (personal communication) have used the scale as a teaching tool with families. Knowledge about grouped behaviors in the scale reportedly helped families to anticipate progressive losses in psychomotor and functional areas as well as cognitive impairment.

PSYCHOMETRIC PROPERTIES: Patients ($N = 16$) were independently rated, on two occasions 10 days apart, by six multidisciplinary staff members at a day hospital. The mean for correlations of agreements between the 15 possible pairs of raters and for both occasions was 0.90. "Correlations within pairs for each of the eight specific items were comparable to those for total scores" (Haycox, 1984, p. 23), ranging between 0.87 and 0.96. The correlation for test-retest reliability was 0.97. Scores on the HDBS were correlated with scores on the Blessed Dementia Scale (see entry in this book; $r = 0.61$, $p < 0.01$).

PROCEDURE: The scale is completed by an observer who knows the subject. The rater may ask family members to give information about behaviors that occur at home. The rater underlines the behaviors that apply and then circles the score that indicates the person's current status for the category.

SAMPLE ITEMS: Three of seven items for eating and nutrition:

"Needs prompting to eat, history of weight loss, burns pots"; "Needs food cut up, wanders from table, can't cook at all"; and "Improper use of utensils, uses fingers, slight weight gain" (Haycox, 1984, p. 24).

SCORING: Normal behavior in a category is scored 0. Scores for deficit behaviors range from 1 to 6. Total scores for the HDBS range from 0 to 48, with higher scores indicating more deficit.

SOURCE: The scale is reprinted in Haycox (1984).

REFERENCES

Haycox, J. (1984). A simple, reliable clinical behavioral scale for assessing demented patients. *Journal of Clinical Psychiatry, 45,* 23-24.

Rosswurm, M. A. (1989). Assessment of perceptual processing deficits in persons with Alzheimer's disease. *Western Journal of Nursing Research, 11,* 458-468.

HEALTH-SPECIFIC FAMILY COPING INDEX (HSFCI)

AUTHORS: Thomas Choi, LaVohn Josten, and Mary Lou Christensen
ADDRESS: LaVohn E. Josten, PhD, RN
            School of Nursing, University of Minnesota
            6-101 Unit F, 308 Harvard Street Southeast
            Minneapolis, MN 55455

DESCRIPTION: The Health-Specific Family Coping Index (HSFCI; Choi, Josten, & Christensen, 1983) was modified and adapted from the Richmond/Hopkins Visiting Nurses Association Family Coping Index developed by Freeman and Lowe (1963). The index is used to rate families in nine domains: "physical independence, therapeutic competence, knowledge of health condition, application of principles of general hygiene, health care attitude, emotional competence, family living patterns, physical environment, and use of community resources" (Choi et al., 1983, p. 1276).

PSYCHOMETRIC PROPERTIES: Christensen, Josten, and Choi (1983) developed an operations manual for the HSFCI to clarify the instructions provided by the original authors. They differentiated the nine domains of the HSFCI more clearly and defined each level of coping to facilitate the reliability of ratings (Choi et al., 1983, p. 1275). In a validation study, 50 public health nurses rated seven vignettes of family coping based on actual cases. A General Aptitude Family Coping Index (GAFCI) constructed for the study was designed by experts to "gauge the family's potential for coping as stressful life events occur" (p. 1275). The HSFCI and the GAFCI were significantly correlated (0.94; p. 1276). The new form for the HSFCI explained more of the variance (83%) than the original version did (59%; p. 1276). Internal consistency (coefficient alpha) for the HSFCI ranged between 0.97 and 0.99 (p. 1276).

PROCEDURE: The assessment to complete each of the nine subscales is made using the definitions provided in the manual. Coping examples are provided with the definition for each rating.

SAMPLE ITEM: Physical Environment.

1 = Physical environment is very hazardous.

2 = Physical environment is dominated by hazards.

3 = Moderate environmental hazards exist, but the family can compensate for them.

4 = Environment is free of hazards, but contains few factors that enhance the quality of life.

5 = Environment is free of hazards and promotes family members' physical and emotional well-being. (Christensen et al., 1983, pp. 24-25)

SCORING: For each of the nine subscales, the range of scores is 1 to 5. A summary score is obtained by adding the subscale scores; therefore, the range for total raw HSFCI score is 9 to 45. Investigators and/or clinicians may calculate a "percentage-of-functioning" score from HSFCI ratings as estimates of change in families before and after nursing interventions. To get the percentage-of-functioning score, the total raw score is divided by 45, and multiplied by 100 (Christensen et al., 1983, p. 28).

SOURCE: The HSFCI instrument and its manual are available from Professor Josten. The GAFCI is reprinted in Choi et al. (1983).

REFERENCES

Choi, T., Josten, L., & Christensen, M. L. (1983). Health-specific family coping index for non-institutional care. *American Journal of Public Health, 73,* 1275-1277.

Christensen, M. L., Josten, L., & Choi, T. (1983). *Health-Specific Family Coping Index.* (Available from Mary Lou Christensen, Ramsey County Public Health Nursing Service, 910 American Center Building, 150 East Kellogg Boulevard, St. Paul, MN 55101)

Freeman, R. B., & Lowe, M. (1963). A method for appraising family public health nursing need. *American Journal of Public Health, 53,* 47-52.

HEARING HANDICAP INVENTORY FOR THE ELDERLY (HHIE)

AUTHORS: Ira M. Ventry and Barbara E. Weinstein
ADDRESS: Barbara E. Weinstein, PhD
             Lehman College, CUNY
             Bedford Park Boulevard West
             Bronx, NY 10468

DESCRIPTION: The Hearing Handicap Inventory for the Elderly (HHIE) is a 25-item self-assessment scale (Ventry & Weinstein, 1982). The HHIE is not a hearing test per se; rather, it is a tool used to "assess the effects of hearing impairment on the emotional and social adjustment of elderly people" (p. 128). The authors believe that "hearing impairment is only one facet of handicap and that evaluation of handicap requires more information than that provided by audiometry alone" (p. 128). The HHIE, which was intended for use with noninstitutionalized elderly persons, has two subscales: an emotional subscale with 13 items and a social/situational subscale with 12 items.

PSYCHOMETRIC PROPERTIES: A team of expert audiologists generated preliminary items, which were revised after pilot studies. To standardize the HHIE, the authors administered it to 100 older persons with a range of hearing impairments. Members of the sample were like persons "routinely serviced by speech and hearing centers in large urban communities" (Ventry & Weinstein, 1982, p. 130). Reliability of the HHIE was estimated with Cronbach's alpha. For the total scale and subscales, alphas ranged between 0.88 and 0.95. There was a moderate correlation between HHIE scores and increasing hearing impairment ($r = 0.61$; p. 131). Some persons with "significant" impairment, however, had low HHIE scores, and some with minimal loss had high HHIE scores (p. 131). The authors interpreted this variability as supporting the construct validity of the scale (p. 133). Newman and Weinstein (1989) demonstrated test-retest reliability ($N = 19$) using a face-to-face format initially, followed by a paper-and-pencil format 6 weeks later. Correlation coefficients for total scale and subscales ranged from 0.91 to 0.94. An adaptation of the HHIE for younger adults (HHIA; Newman, Weinstein, Jacobson, & Hug, 1991) and a form for spouses of hearing impaired persons (HHIE-SP; Newman & Weinstein, 1986) have also been published. Weinstein (1986) also developed a 10-item version (HHIE-S) of the HHIE that has been used for screening. Both the original (Newman & Weinstein, 1988) and the shortened version (Newman, Jacobson, Hug, Weinstein, & Malinoff, 1991) have been used to quantify the benefit of hearing aid placement.

PROCEDURE: The HHIE was designed to be administered "face to face" in an interview. It is also suitable as a paper-and-pencil test. Instructions explain its purpose and advise the respondent: "Do not skip a question if you avoid a situation because of your hearing problem" (Ventry & Weinstein, 1982, p. 134). If subjects use a hearing aid, answers should refer to their hearing "without the aid." Administration takes about 10 minutes.

SAMPLE ITEMS:

S-1. Does a hearing problem cause you to use the phone less often than you would like?

E-2. Does a hearing problem cause you to feel embarrassed when meeting new people? (Ventry & Weinstein, 1982, p. 134)

SCORING: Scores range from 0 to 100. Respondents rate items *yes* (4), *sometimes* (2), or *no* (0). On the basis of their data, the authors interpreted "a score of 18% or greater as suggesting a self-perceived handicap" (Ventry & Weinstein, 1982, p. 133).

SOURCE: A copy of the instrument appears as an appendix to Ventry and Weinstein (1982). Other versions of the instrument are in Newman, Weinstein, et al. (1991), Newman and Weinstein (1986), and Newman, Jacobson, et al. (1991).

REFERENCES

Newman, C. W., Jacobson, G. P., Hug, G. A., Weinstein, B. E., & Malinoff, R. L. (1991). Practical method for quantifying hearing aid benefit in older adults. *Journal of the American Academy of Audiology, 2,* 70-75.

Newman, C. W., & Weinstein, B. E. (1986). Judgments of perceived hearing handicap by hearing-impaired elderly men and their spouses. *Journal of the Academy of Rehabilitation Audiology, 19,* 109-115.

Newman, C. W., & Weinstein, B. E. (1988). The Hearing Handicap Inventory for the elderly as a measure of hearing aid benefit. *Ear and Hearing, 9,* 81-85.

Newman, C. W., & Weinstein, B. E. (1989). Test-retest reliability of the Hearing Handicap Inventory for the elderly using two administration approaches. *Ear and Hearing, 10,* 190-191.

Newman, C. W., Weinstein, B. E., Jacobson, G. P., & Hug, G. A. (1991). Test-retest reliability of the Hearing Handicap Inventory for adults. *Ear and Hearing, 12,* 355-357.

Ventry, I. M., & Weinstein, B. E. (1982). The Hearing Handicap Inventory for the elderly: A new tool. *Ear and Hearing, 3,* 128-134.

Weinstein, B. E. (1986). Validity of a screening protocol for identifying elderly people with hearing problems. *American Speech and Hearing Association, 28*(5), 41-45.

HERTH HOPE SCALE (HHS)

AUTHOR: Kaye A. Herth

ADDRESS: Kaye A. Herth
            Professor and Chair, Department of Nursing
            Georgia Southern University
            Landrum Box 8158
            Statesboro, GA 30460-8158

DESCRIPTION: The Herth Hope Scale (HHS) is a 30-item instrument designed to "capture the multidimensionality of hope" (Herth, 1991, p. 41) and to measure the construct in both well and ill adults (Herth, 1995). There are three subscales for the instrument: (a) temporality and future, (b) positive readiness and expectancy, and (c) interconnectedness. The scale has been printed in large type. Items were developed for a sixth-grade reading level.

PSYCHOMETRIC PROPERTIES: The instrument was pretested and piloted with cancer patients. Four expert judges from various disciplines evaluated the content for HHS items. The author tested the scale with several ethnically diverse samples of well adults, including elderly persons. Mean hope scores for well adults ($n = 185$) were 80, with a range between 60 and 90. For a sample of "community elderly" ($n = 40$), the mean was 72, with a range between 52 and 88. Cancer patients' hope scores were lower. The possibility that scores are influenced by social desirability needs further study (Herth, 1991). Test-retest ($n = 40$) at 3-week intervals supported reliability. Negative correlations with a hopelessness scale demonstrated validity. Three factors were supported with data from all samples, with appropriate alpha coefficients, such as those for a bereaved elderly sample ($n = 75$) at 0.91, 0.90, and 0.87. Alpha coefficients for the total scores were also high.

PROCEDURE: The respondent has four possible choices for each of the 30 items on the scale: *never applies to me, seldom applies to me, sometimes applies to me,* or *often applies to me.*

SAMPLE ITEMS: "I have deep inner strength," "I believe that each day has potential," and "I am immobilized by fears and doubts" (Herth, 1991, p. 47).

SCORING: Scores for each item (0, 1, 2, or 3) are summed for both the subscales and the total scale. Six negatively phrased items are scored in reverse. Total scores may range from 0 to 90; higher scores are associated with greater hope.

SOURCE: Copies of the HHS are available from the author, who holds a copyright. The instrument has been translated into Spanish and Thai (Herth, 1995). Herth has also developed a 12-item adapted version of the HHS, the Herth Hope Index (HHI), designed for assessment of hope in clinical settings (Herth, 1992). The HHI has been translated into Swedish and Chinese.

REFERENCES

Herth, K. (1991). Development and refinement of an instrument to measure hope. *Scholarly Inquiry for Nursing Practice, 5,* 39-51.

Herth, K. (1992). Abbreviated instrument to measure hope: Development and psychometric evaluation. *Journal of Advanced Nursing, 17,* 1251-1259.

Herth, K. (1995). Critique of existing measures. In C. J. Farran, K. A. Herth, & J. M. Popovich (Eds.), *Hope and hopelessness: Critical clinical constructs* (pp. 43-76). Thousand Oaks, CA: Sage.

INDEX OF INDEPENDENCE IN ACTIVITIES OF DAILY LIVING (INDEXADL)

AUTHORS: Sidney Katz and Associates

DESCRIPTION: The Index of Independence in Activities of Daily Living (INDEXADL) was developed "to study results of treatment and prognosis in the elderly and chronically ill" (Katz, Ford, Quick, Moskowitz, Jackson, & Jaffe, 1963, p. 914). An observer using responses to the index can summarize a subject's performance in bathing, dressing, toileting, transferring, continence, and feeding. The index permits ranking of subjects according to the adequacy of their performance and focuses on the actual assistance given to the person rather than his or her potential or ability (Katz & Akpom, 1976, p. 497). After completing the evaluation forms, the observer applies definitions of independence and dependence for each ADL and assigns one of the following grades:

A   = Independent in feeding, continence, transferring, going to toilet, dressing and bathing

B   = Independent in all but one of these functions

C   = Independent in all but bathing and one additional function

D   = Independent in all but bathing, dressing, and one additional function

E   = Independent in all but bathing, dressing, going to toilet, and one additional function

F   = Independent in all but bathing, dressing, going to toilet, transferring, and one additional function

G   = Dependent in all six functions

Other = Dependent in at least two functions, but not classifiable as C, D, E, or F (Katz et al., 1963, p. 915)

The authors found that "the order of recovery of index functions in disabled patients is remarkably similar to the order of development of primary functions in children" (p. 914).

PSYCHOMETRIC PROPERTIES: Simultaneous independent observations were made to check "degree of reliability," with differences between observers occurring "once in 20 evaluations or less frequently" (Katz et al., 1963, p. 915). INDEXADL grades assigned to patients were related to concurrent assistance needed, as well as to predictions of future needs for assistance. For example, patients graded B or C received sporadic assistance, while those graded D through G received assistance more frequently. Of 154 evaluated 1 year after illness onset, those initially graded B or C were less likely to have nonfamily home attendants than those graded D through G.

PROCEDURE: The observer may ask the subject to show him or her "(1) the bathroom, and (2) medications in another room (or a meaningful substitute object)" (p. 915). These instructions create opportunities for observation of performance to corroborate information gathered verbally. The observer uses the evaluation form as a guide to rate "the most dependent degree of performance" (Katz, Downs, Cash, & Grotz, 1970, p. 22) during the 2-week period preceding the evaluation. Data gathered on the form are later converted to one of the INDEXADL grades, using specific criteria. Restrictions of independence may occasionally be imposed in a particular environment. For example, there may be a policy at a nursing home that staff must supervise tub baths. Because independence for the index means "without supervision, direction or active personal assistance except as specifically noted" (Katz et al., 1963, p. 915), observations of supervision might affect an independence rating.

SAMPLE ITEM: Transfer Item (from evaluation form; Katz et al., 1970): "Moves in or out of bed as well as in and out of chair without assistance; may be using object for support such as cane or walker," "Moves in or out of bed or chair with assistance," or "Doesn't get out of bed" (p. 21). Transfer Item (from grading form; Katz et al., 1970): "Independent: moves in and out of bed independently and moves in and out of chair independently (may or may not be using mechanical supports)" and "Dependent: assistance in moving in and out of bed and/or chair; does not perform one or more transfers" (p. 23).

SCORING: The letter grades of the INDEXADL are categorical ratings. A modified numerical form of ordinal grading can eliminate the "other" category. Grades in this format stand for the number of activities of daily living in which the individual is dependent, from 0 to 6. This scoring is possible because there is an "inherent consistency" in the "hierarchically ordered profiles" summarized by the index (Katz & Akpom, 1976, p. 497).

SOURCE: Copies of the instrument and its evaluation forms appear in Katz et al. (1963, 1970) and Katz and Akpom (1976).

REFERENCES

Katz, S., & Akpom, C. A. (1976). A measure of primary sociobiological functions. *International Journal of Health Services, 6,* 493-508.

Katz, S., Downs, T. D., Cash, H. R., & Grotz, R. C. (1970). Progress in development in the Index of ADL. *Gerontologist, 10,* 20-30.

Katz, S., Ford, A. B., Quick, D. M., Moskowitz, R. W., Jackson, B., & Jaffe, M. W. (1963). Studies of illness in the aged. The index of ADL: A standardized measure of biological and psychological function. *Journal of the American Medical Association, 185,* 914-919.

INTERPERSONAL RELATIONSHIP INVENTORY (IPRI)

AUTHOR: Virginia P. Tilden
ADDRESS: Virginia P. Tilden, RN, DNSc
            School of Nursing, Oregon Health Sciences University
            3181 S.W. Sam Jackson Park Road, SN-ORD
            Portland, OR 97201-3098

DESCRIPTION: The Tilden Interpersonal Relationship Inventory (IPRI) is a measure of three elements of interpersonal relationships known to affect health: social support, conflict, and reciprocity. Developed for use with community-dwelling samples, the IPRI (long form) consists of 39 items: 22 refer to perceived sentiments, and 17 tap frequency of behavior. The IPRI has been used in at least 19 studies (Tilden, Hirsch, & Nelson, 1994) with diverse adult samples, including elderly hospitalized persons and caregivers of persons with Alzheimer's disease.

PSYCHOMETRIC PROPERTIES: To ensure that items would be based on actual experience, items were developed from content analyses of interviews with community-based and hospitalized adults and further validated by experts' judgments (Tilden, Nelson, & May, 1990b). Initial psychometric evaluations with a total of 868 subjects were conducted in six separate validity studies (Tilden, Nelson, & May, 1990a). "Compelling" evidence for construct validity of the Social Support and Conflict subscales and "moderate" evidence for the Reciprocity subscale were reported. Methods to estimate construct validity included theory testing, known groups, factor analysis, and multitrait-multimethod techniques (Tilden et al., 1994). In initial testing, 2-week test-retest reliability was 0.91 for social support, 0.84 for reciprocity, and 0.81 for conflict (Tilden et al., 1990a, p. 338). Internal consistency has ranged between 0.80 and 0.95 for social support, 0.70 and 0.89 for reciprocity, and 0.70 and 0.92 for conflict (Tilden et al., 1994). The measure has been translated into Spanish and French. With the permission of the author, some investigators have modified items to fit specific situations. Use of IPRI items with residents of long-term care facilities might require such modification.

PROCEDURE: The IPRI reportedly takes 10 to 15 minutes to complete. In addition to rating 39 items on Likert scales, respondents also list people who are important to them and state the nature of the relationship. In addition to demographic questions (age, gender, marital status, education, race/ethnicity, employment), respondents also answer two questions about the structures of their relationships: "How many of your close relatives live within 50 miles of you?" and "How many people live with you in your household?" The second of the two is an example of an item that would need to be modified for a long-term care resident sample. The respondent completes the tool with paper and pencil.

SAMPLE ITEM: "If I need help, all I have to do is ask" (Tilden, 1993).

SCORING: The Social Support, Conflict, and Reciprocity subscale scores are designed to be used separately, not combined. Scores for the subscales range between 13 and 65.

SOURCE: The instruments and scoring information for both the long and short forms of the IPRI are available from the author.

REFERENCES

Tilden, V. P. (1993). *The Interpersonal Relationship Inventory.* (Available from the author at address listed above)

Tilden, V. P., Hirsch, A. M., & Nelson, C. A. (1994). The Interpersonal Relationship Inventory: Continued psychometric evaluation. *Journal of Nursing Measurement, 2,* 63-78.

Tilden, V. P., Nelson, C. A., & May, B. A. (1990a). The Interpersonal Relationship Inventory: Development and psychometric characteristics. *Nursing Research, 39,* 337-343.

Tilden, V. P., Nelson, C. A., & May, B. A. (1990b). Use of qualitative methods to enhance content validity. *Nursing Research, 39,* 172-175.

JALOWIEC COPING SCALE (JCS)

AUTHOR: Anne Jalowiec
ADDRESS: Anne Jalowiec, RN, PhD
             School of Nursing, Bldg. 131N, Room 21
             Loyola Medical Center
             2160 South First Avenue
             Maywood, IL 60153

DESCRIPTION: The Jalowiec Coping Scale (JCS) is a questionnaire about the use and effectiveness of specific coping strategies. An early version of the instrument was widely used with diverse groups. Scale items were drawn from a broad literature and a wide empirical base. Jalowiec revised her original 40-item JCS, created in 1977 (Jalowiec, 1979) to increase the instrument's precision and utility. The revised 60-item version, created in 1987 (Jalowiec, 1988) reflects eight possible coping styles: confrontive, evasive, optimistic, fatalistic, emotive, palliative, supportant, and self-reliant.

PSYCHOMETRIC PROPERTIES: The psychometric assessment of the 1977 instrument from which the 1987 version was derived showed satisfactory standards for reliability. Test-retest coefficients were 0.79 ($N = 28$) and 0.78 ($N = 30$; Jalowiec, Murphy, & Powers, 1984, p. 158). Results of factor analysis ($N = 141$) for the 1977 version showed that coping behavior was a multidimensional rather than a unidimensional construct (p. 160). For the 1987 version, the mean for alpha coefficients of "total use" scores in 12 studies was 0.86 (range 0.64 to 0.97). The mean for alpha coefficients of "total effectiveness" scores in the same studies was 0.90 (range 0.84 to 0.96). In a study of cardiac transplant patients, the instrument and its subscales were stable over time. Construct validity was supported by a study in which 25 nurse researchers classified each of the 60 items into one or more of the eight subscale categories. Percentages of agreement between the raters and the author ranged from 54% to 94% (Jalowiec, 1988).

PROCEDURE: The investigator or clinician specifies the focal stress in a space on the front of the scale booklet. In Part A of the tool, the respondent rates the frequency for his or her use of a coping strategy described in the item on a 4-point scale from *never used* (0) to *used often* (3). If the strategy has been used, the subject answers Part B, in which the extent to which the strategy has been helpful is rated on another 4-point scale, from *not helpful* (0) to *very helpful* (3).

SAMPLE ITEMS: "Set up a plan of action" and "Slept more than usual" (Jalowiec, 1988).

SCORING: The scale yields several different kinds of scores. The "overall use" score is the sum of ratings for use for all items. The "overall effectiveness" score is the sum of ratings for effectiveness for all items. Scores may also be computed for each of the eight coping styles, for a combined use multiplied by effectiveness score, and for a "relative" score that takes all coping styles into consideration. Choice of scoring protocols will depend on the nature of the inquiry or practice (Jalowiec, 1988). Detailed instructions about computation of scores are available from the author.

SOURCE: The revised version of the scale and related materials (Jalowiec, 1988) are available from the author, who holds the copyright. There are major differences between the original scale (Jalowiec, 1979) and its revision. Many articles about studies in which the scale was used refer to the original scale.

REFERENCES

Jalowiec, A. (1979). *Stress and coping in hypertensive and emergency room patients.* Unpublished master's thesis, University of Illinois, Chicago.

Jalowiec, A. (1988). *The Jalowiec Coping Scale (Revised Version).* (Available from the author at address listed above)

Jalowiec, A., Murphy, S. P., & Powers, M. J. (1984). Psychometric assessment of the Jalowiec Coping Scale. *Nursing Research, 33,* 157-161.

KARNOFSKY PERFORMANCE STATUS (KPS)

AUTHORS: David A. Karnofsky, Walter H. Abelmann,
            Lloyd F. Craver, and Joseph H. Burchenal

DESCRIPTION: The Karnofsky Performance Status (KPS) scale is a measure of functional status for rating ability to carry on normal activities and degree of dependence on help and nursing care (Karnofsky, Abelmann, Craver, & Burchenal, 1948, p. 635). It provides a global score that has been used as an outcome measure and an eligibility criterion for selecting stratified clinical samples. The scale has 11 categories and scores from 0 to 100 in increments of 10. There are descriptions of function and quality of life corresponding to each ordinal rating. In addition, three categories of performance anchor the 100%, 70%, and 40% intervals. Descriptions range from "normal; no complaints; no evidence of disease," for 100%, to "moribund; fatal processes progressing rapidly" for 10%. Zero signifies death (Karnofsky et al., 1948, p. 635). The KPS has been widely used for patients with cancer and end-stage renal disease; recently it has been suggested for use with heart patients (O'Brien, Buxton, & Patterson, 1993), and it has been seen as an effective proxy score for the health and functional status of geriatric patients (Crooks, Waller, & Smith, 1991).

PSYCHOMETRIC PROPERTIES: The initial work with this scale in the 1940s was clinically focused. It was used to evaluate the effects of treatments for cancer. Efforts to refine the KPS to increase its effectiveness for research and clinical decision making have continued. Mor, Laliberte, Morris, and Weimann (1984) suggested training raters to gain high levels of reliability. They trained interviewers in an intensive program of instruction, testing, field experience, and retesting. Following the training, interrater reliability for ratings of patient narratives made by 47 raters was 0.97. In the Mor et al. (1984) study of hospice patients ($N = 685$), KPS scores were compared with activities of daily living (ADL) ratings. The investigators found that the proportion of patients able to function independently increased as the KPS score increased (p. 2004). Validity was further supported by significant correspondence between KPS ratings, scores for a severity index, and an independently rated physical quality of life score derived for the study (p. 2005). Predictive validity for the KPS was substantiated with the hospice sample by a significant relationship between KPS and days of survival (p. 2006). Crooks et al. (1991) investigated the use of the KPS for geriatric outpatients and found the instrument "highly predictive of hospitalizations, survival days, community residence and institutionalization, performing better or equally well as a predictor of patient outcomes as the ADL and IADL" (p. M142).

PROCEDURE: Following orientation and practice sessions with the instrument, the observer rates performance status, using data gathered in interviews with patients and/or caregivers and/or from records.

SAMPLE ITEMS: "Unable to work. Able to live at home, care for most personal needs. A varying amount of assistance is needed" and "Cares for self. Unable to carry on normal activity or do active work" (Karnofsky et al., 1948, p. 635).

SCORING: The score is the percentage rated, from 100% through 10% in increments of 10, or the corresponding numeral, from 10 to 1.

SOURCE: The instrument is reprinted in Karnofsky et al. (1948) and Mor et al. (1984). Columbia University Press holds the copyright for the KPS.

REFERENCES

Crooks, V., Waller, S., & Smith, T. (1991). The use of the Karnofsky Performance Scale in determining outcomes and risk in geriatric outpatients. *Journal of Gerontology: Medical Sciences, 46,* M139-M144.

Karnofsky, D. A., Abelmann, W. H., Craver, L. F., & Burchenal, J. H. (1948). The use of the nitrogen mustards in the palliative treatment of carcinoma. *Cancer, 1,* 634-656.

Mor, V., Laliberte, L., Morris, J. N., & Weimann, M. (1984). The Karnofsky Performance Status Scale: An examination of its reliability and validity in a research setting. *Cancer, 53,* 2002-2007.

O'Brien, B. J., Buxton, M. J., & Patterson, D. L. (1993). Relationship between functional status and health-related quality-of-life after myocardial infarction. *Medical Care, 31,* 950-955.

KAYSER-JONES BRIEF ORAL HEALTH STATUS EXAMINATION (BOHSE)

AUTHOR: Jeanie Kayser-Jones
ADDRESS: Jeanie Kayser-Jones, RN, PhD
           University of California, San Francisco
           Department of Physiological Nursing, Box 0610
           San Francisco, CA 94143

DESCRIPTION: The Kayser-Jones Brief Oral Health Status Examination (BOHSE) is an instrument designed to be used by nursing personnel to assess the oral health of nursing home residents. The instrument is not intended as a diagnostic tool; rather, it is a method to "assist dentists by bringing problems to their attention in a timely fashion" (Kayser-Jones, Bird, Paul, Long, & Schell, 1995, p. 823). The areas of oral health covered by the assessment include the "lymph nodes, lips, tongue, tissue inside the cheek, floor and roof of the mouth, gums, saliva, condition of natural and/or artificial teeth, pairs of teeth in chewing position and oral cleanliness" (p. 823).

PSYCHOMETRIC PROPERTIES: The instrument, which was based on recommendations of the American Dental Society, was developed from the oral health literature, with consultation from members of a dental school faculty. Kayser-Jones et al. (1995) found that all levels of nursing staff could be instructed to assess the oral health of nursing home residents. Their study was conducted in one long-term care facility with 100 residents. Mean age for residents was 82 years; 48% of the sample were assessed as "severely impaired." The residents were examined both by dentists and by registered nurses (RNs), licensed vocational nurses (LVNs), and nurse's aides (NAs) who had been trained in a continuing education program. Interrater reliability coefficients for ratings of dentists and other raters, all significant at 0.001, were 0.63 for dentists and RNs, 0.68 for dentists and LVNs, and 0.47 for dentists and NAs (p. 818). Test-retest reliability was estimated with exams of one third of the sample, with correlations ranging between 0.79 and 0.88. Mean total BOHSE scores for the sample ranged between 3.75 and 5.06 (p. 819).

PROCEDURE: The subject sits in bed or in a chair. The following equipment is needed: "tongue blades, a hand-held light, gauze squares, and disposable gloves" (Kayser-Jones et al., 1995, p. 818). The examiner, who should be trained for the process, follows the guidelines in the "Measurement" column of the instrument. For example, for the item "Gums between teeth and/or under artificial teeth," the instruction is: "Gently press gums with tip of tongue blade" (p. 823). The exam takes between 5 and 20 minutes to complete. Mean exam time for RNs was 7.4 minutes (p. 818).

SAMPLE ITEM: Condition of Natural Teeth:

0 = No decayed or broken teeth/roots.
1 = 1 to 3 decayed or broken teeth/roots.
2 = 4 or more decayed or broken teeth/roots; fewer than 4 teeth in jaw (Kayser-Jones et al., 1995, p. 823). Note: Under Conditions 1 and 2 in this item, the individual would be immediately referred to a dentist.

SCORING: Each item has "three descriptors" that allow rating on a 3-point scale, from 0 to 2. The 0 rating is at the healthy end of the scale. Total BOHSE scores range between 0 and 20.

SOURCE: The instrument is reprinted in Kayser-Jones et al. (1995). It is copyrighted. Clinicians and researchers who wish to use the BOHSE will need to write to Dr. Kayser-Jones to obtain permission.

REFERENCE

Kayser-Jones, J., Bird, W. F., Paul, S. M., Long, L., & Schell, E. S. (1995). An instrument to assess the oral health status of nursing home residents. *Gerontologist, 35,* 814-824.

KRANTZ HEALTH OPINION SURVEY (HOS)

AUTHOR: David S. Krantz
ADDRESS: Professor David S. Krantz
              Uniformed Services University of the Health Sciences
              4301 Jones Bridge Road
              Bethesda, MD 20814-4799

DESCRIPTION: The Krantz Health Opinion Survey (HOS) is a 16-item forced-choice questionnaire designed to elicit preferences for an active, informed stance versus a relatively inactive and trusting patient role in the health care process (Krantz, Baum, & Wideman, 1980, p. 979). The HOS has two subscales, an Information subscale with seven items (HOS-I) and a Behavioral Involvement subscale with nine items (HOS-BI).

PSYCHOMETRIC PROPERTIES: With several samples of college under-graduates, reliability coefficients for total HOS scores and subscale scores ranged between 0.74 and 0.77. Test-retest reliabilities ranged between 0.59 and 0.74. The two subscales of the instrument correlated only slightly with each other. Validity was supported when scores on the HOS discriminated between high self-care groups and a general student population. Students with lower HOS-BI scores were more likely to visit a student clinic. Krantz et al. (1980) demonstrated a "linear negative relationship to reported use of clinic facilities" (p. 983) for both HOS and HOS-BI scores. Total HOS scores and HOS-BI scores were also associated with self-diagnosis. High total HOS and HOS-I scores were associated with more inquisitiveness. There was a positive linear relationship between the number of questions asked of a health care worker and total HOS and HOS-I scores. Smith, Wallston, Wallston, Forsberg, and King (1984) studied two samples of adults ($N = 243$) with average ages of 49.67 and 44.2 and found that the HOS-I enabled them to discriminate between groups who wanted or did not want control of health care processes. Alpha coefficients for these samples for the HOS-I ranged between 0.73 and 0.78 and for the HOS-BI ranged between 0.78 and 0.83. Another investigator (Dennis, 1987) who used the HOS with a hospitalized sample (age range = 24 to 75 years) found evidence of predictive validity for the HOS (p. 152).

PROCEDURE: Respondents are informed that there are no right or wrong answers to the survey. They are asked to circle a response (*agree* or *disagree*) that comes closest to what they believe about each of the 16 items, even if they find that they cannot completely agree or disagree with the statement.

SAMPLE HOS-I ITEM: "I usually ask the doctor or nurse lots of questions about the procedures during a medical exam" (Krantz et al., 1980, p. 980).

SAMPLE HOS-BI ITEM: "It's almost always better to seek professional help than to try to treat yourself" (Krantz et al., 1980, p. 980).

SCORING: The instrument yields a total score and two subscores. Higher scores "represent favorable attitudes toward self-directed or informed treatment" (Krantz et al., 1980, p. 980). Some items on the scale are worded negatively and are therefore scored in reverse.

SOURCE: A copy of the HOS and instructions for its administration are available from the author. The items are listed in Krantz et al. (1980).

REFERENCES

Dennis, K. E. (1987). Dimensions of client control. *Nursing Research, 36,* 151-156.
Krantz, D. S., Baum, A., & Wideman, M. V. (1980). Assessment of preferences for self-treatment and information in health care. *Journal of Personality and Social Psychology, 39,* 977-990.
Smith, R. A., Wallston, B. S., Wallston, K. A., Forsberg, P. R., & King, J. E. (1984). Measuring desire for control in health care. *Journal of Personality and Social Psychology, 47,* 415-427.

McGILL PAIN QUESTIONNAIRE (MPQ)

AUTHOR: Ronald Melzack
ADDRESS: Dr. Ronald Melzack
            Department of Psychology
            McGill University
            1205 Dr. Penfield Avenue
            Montreal, Quebec H3A 1B1, Canada

DESCRIPTION: Construction of the McGill Pain Questionnaire (MPQ) was based on the assumption that measuring pain involved more than mere gauging of intensity. According to Katz and Melzack (1992), there are "three major psychological dimensions of pain: sensory-discriminative, motivational-affective, and cognitive-evaluative" (p. 230). The MPQ was designed to yield quantitative information about pain by generating answers to four questions: "1) Where is the pain? 2) What does it feel like? 3) How does it change with time? 4) How strong is it?" (Melzack, 1975, p. 280). The corresponding components of the MPQ (Katz & Melzack, 1992) are (a) line drawings of a human body, (b) a list of 78 pain descriptors in 20 subclasses, (c) words to elicit temporal information, and (d) a scale to rate present intensity from 1 (*mild*) to 5 (*excruciating*) (p. 234). There are at least five versions of the MPQ (Wilkie, Savedra, Holzemer, Tesler, & Paul, 1990), including a shortened version (Melzack, 1987). The tool has been translated into many languages and adapted by clinicians and researchers for specific groups.

PSYCHOMETRIC PROPERTIES: The initial work to develop the MPQ involved gathering words describing pain from the clinical literature. Following testing, the words were categorized into four major groups (sensory, affective, evaluative, and miscellaneous) and 20 subclasses (Melzack, 1975). Groups of physicians, patients, and students assigned intensity values to the words and were in agreement about rankings (p. 278). Wilkie et al. (1990) conducted a meta-analytic study to estimate normative means for MPQ scores. They used data from 51 studies in which the MPQ was used with samples totaling 3,624 persons.

PROCEDURE: The standard MPQ is printed on one page. Administration is reported to take 5 to 10 minutes (Melzack, 1987) or 15 to 30 minutes (McGuire, 1984) and requires "intense concentration from respondents" (p. 156). There is no manual for the tool, but instructions are clear in Melzack (1975). The MPQ may be administered orally or in a written format. For greatest reliability, Melzack recommended verbal administration. The list of pain descriptors is read aloud to respondents, using an unhurried pace. Respondents are instructed to select *only* those words that describe their feelings and sensations at the time of administration. Words may be defined or reread as needed. Subjects mark the line drawings, showing areas where they feel pain and indicating whether it is felt internally ("I") or externally ("E") or both ("EI"). Areas that can "trigger pain when pressure is applied" are marked with an X (Melzack, 1975, p. 298).

SAMPLE ITEM: Subclass 5 of pain descriptors: "pinching, pressing, gnawing, cramping, crushing" (Melzack, 1975, p. 281).

SCORING: Three main pain scores may be derived from data gathered with the MPQ. The Pain Rating Index (PRI) is based on the ranked values for pain descriptors chosen. The words representing pain in each subclass are assigned values. PRIs may be computed for each of the four major categories: sensory (Subclasses 1-10), affective (Subclasses 11-15), evaluative (Subclass 16), and miscellaneous (Subclasses 17-20). The total PRI is the sum of the values of descriptors chosen in all categories. The number of words chosen (NWC) is another quantitative measure. The present pain intensity (PPI) at the time of administration is another pain indicator that can be handled statistically. Noting about the PRI that "the subscale scores contribute little beyond what is measured by the total score," Turk, Rudy, and Salovey (1985) suggested that "the total score of the PRI appears to be the most appropriate score to use" (p. 394). Other methods of scoring using weighted rank values have also been reported (Katz & Melzack, 1992, p. 237).

SOURCE: Both standard and short forms of the MPQ are reprinted in Katz and Melzack (1992). In Melzack (1975), there are scoring instructions and two other formats of the MPQ.

REFERENCES

Katz, J., & Melzack, R. (1992). Measure of pain. *Anesthesiology Clinics of North America, 10,* 229-246.

McGuire, D. B. (1984). The measurement of clinical pain. *Nursing Research, 33,* 152-156.

Melzack, R. (1975). The McGill Pain Questionnaire: Major properties and scoring methods. *Pain, 1,* 277-299.

Melzack, R. (1987). The short-form McGill Pain Questionnaire. *Pain, 30,* 191-197.

Turk, D. C., Rudy, T. E., & Salovey, P. (1985). The McGill Pain Questionnaire reconsidered: Confirming the factor structure and examining appropriate uses. *Pain, 21,* 385-397.

Wilkie, D. J., Savedra, M. C., Holzemer, W. L., Tesler, M. D., & Paul, S. I. (1990). Use of the McGill Pain Questionnaire to measure pain: A meta-analysis. *Nursing Research, 39,* 36-41.

MEMORIAL UNIVERSITY OF NEWFOUNDLAND SCALE OF HAPPINESS (MUNSH)

AUTHORS: Albert Kozma and Michael J. Stones
ADDRESS: Albert Kozma, PhD
             Gerontology Center
             Memorial University of Newfoundland
             St. John's, Newfoundland A1B 3X9, Canada

DESCRIPTION: The Memorial University of Newfoundland Scale of Happiness (MUNSH) is an instrument designed to measure mental health and psychological well-being for the elderly. Kozma and Stones (1980) chose happiness as the "construct of choice to best represent the mental health concept in psycho-social gerontology" (p. 906). They constructed the MUNSH using new items and items from the Affect Balance Scale (ABS; Bradburn, 1969), the Life Satisfaction Index-Z (LSI-Z; Wood, Wylie, & Sheafor, 1969), and the Philadelphia Geriatric Center Morale Scale Revised (PGC; see entry in this book). Kozma and Stones (1980) stated that happiness "is best assessed by subtracting negative from positive experiences" (p. 911). The 24 MUNSH items comprise 5 for positive affect (PA), 5 for negative affect (NA), 7 for general positive experience (PE), and 7 for general negative experience (NE; p. 908).

PSYCHOMETRIC PROPERTIES: In Phase I of their work, Kozma and Stones (1980) randomly selected elderly participants from three different environments in Newfoundland ($N = 301$). Subjects completed a battery of tests, including the ABS, PGC, and LSI-Z, and items proposed for the MUNSH. To provide a criterion measure, the participants rated subjective happiness on a seven-rung ladder scale for two time periods: "at this moment" and "over the past month." These two ratings were then combined as one measure of "avowed happiness" (AVHT). Items retained for the final version of the MUNSH were those that were significantly correlated with the AVHT. The MUNSH was significantly better at predicting the criterion rating (AVHT) than were the ABS, LSI-Z, or PGC (p. 909). The authors cross-validated the test with a different sample from Newfoundland including urban ($n = 97$), rural ($n = 100$), and institutional ($n = 100$) elders. The same methods were used as for the first study. Internal consistency for the MUNSH (0.85) was higher than it was for the other scales. Test-retest procedures, conducted at intervals of 6 months to 1 year ($n = 55$), showed that the MUNSH (0.70) was more reliable over time than the LSI-Z (0.35), PGC (0.36), or ABS (0.27; p. 911). The MUNSH was revalidated with a sample of Senior Citizen Home residents ($n = 51$) in an urban setting in another province (Kozma & Stones, 1983). Correlations between MUNSH scores and AVHT ratings (0.86) and between nurse judges' ratings of happiness and MUNSH scores (0.50, $p < 0.001$) supported validity (Kozma & Stones, 1983, p. 28). The scale has also been tested with a younger sample of 117 psychiatric patients and a control group of 40 hospital staff member volunteers with age, gender, and education characteristics similar to those of the patients (Kozma, Stones, & Kazarian, 1985). The authors reported three major conclusions from the study: (a) Reliability coefficients for MUNSH scores of younger subjects were comparable to those for older samples (p. 51), (b) MUNSH scores discriminated between the clinical and volunteer groups (p. 53), and (c) "General measures of well-being discriminate between clinical and community samples primarily on the basis of a depression dimension" (p. 53).

PROCEDURE: In a paper-and-pencil format, the subject responds to items that are prefaced by the words "In the past month have you ever felt: . . . ?" The MUNSH may also be administered orally.

SAMPLE ITEMS: "On top of the world (PA)," "Depressed or very unhappy (NA)," "Most of the things I do are boring or monotonous (NE)," and "I am as happy now as I was when I was younger (PE)" (Kozma & Stones, 1980, p. 910).

SCORING: Items are scored 2 for "yes," 0 for "no," and 1 for "I don't know." The total MUNSH score is calculated by the formula: MUNSH Total = (PAs + PEs) – (NAs + NEs) or MUNSH Total = (PA – NA) + (PE – NE).

SOURCE: A copy of the MUNSH is reprinted in Kozma and Stones (1980). However, three items (17, 19, and 23) have now been reworded. The revised instrument is available from the authors.

REFERENCES

Bradburn, N. (1969). *The structure of psychological well-being.* Chicago: Aldine.

Kozma, A., & Stones, M. J. (1980). The measurement of happiness: Development of the Memorial University of Newfoundland Scale of Happiness (MUNSH). *Journal of Gerontology, 35,* 906-912.

Kozma, A., & Stones, M. J. (1983). Re-validation of the Memorial University of Newfoundland Scale of Happiness. *Canadian Journal of Aging, 2*(1), 27-29.

Kozma, A., Stones, M. J., & Kazarian, S. (1985). The usefulness of the MUNSH as a measure of well-being and psychopathology. *Social Indicators Research, 17,* 49-55.

Wood, V., Wylie, M. L., & Sheafor, B. (1969). An analysis of a short self-report measure of life satisfaction: Correlation with rater judgments. *Journal of Gerontology, 24,* 465-469.

MEMORY AND BEHAVIOR PROBLEMS CHECKLIST—1990R (MBPC)

AUTHORS: Steven H. Zarit and Judy M. Zarit

ADDRESS: Gerontology Center
College of Health and Human Development
Pennsylvania State University
240 Henderson Building South
University Park, PA 16802

DESCRIPTION: The Memory and Behavior Problems Checklist—1990R (MBPC) is a 26-item instrument designed "to determine how frequently a dementia patient engages in problematic behaviors, and which problems are especially upsetting for family members" (Zarit & Zarit, 1990, p. 2). Respondents are family members or other persons who know how the person with dementia typically behaves. Scores provide an estimate of the severity of functional behavior problems and do not represent the severity of dementia.

PSYCHOMETRIC PROPERTIES: The 1990R version of this instrument has 26 items drawn from the 64-item Revised Memory and Behavior Problems Checklist (Teri et al., 1990), which in turn was based on an earlier tool. The reliability and validity information available (Zarit, Anthony, & Boutselis, 1987) refers to a 1982 form. Split-half reliability for frequency was 0.65; for caregiver reaction, it was 0.66. Test-retest reliability was estimated at 0.80 for frequency and 0.56 for caregiver reaction. Validity was supported by comparing checklist scores with global estimates of the severity of cognitive impairments in persons with dementia. Correlations ranged from 0.49 to 0.69. Neundorfer (1991), using an earlier 30-item version of the checklist in a study of 60 spouse caregivers, reported alpha coefficients of 0.86 for frequency ratings and 0.94 for ratings of reactions. She termed reactions of caregivers "appraisal of stress" and found that it was a significant predictor of depression and anxiety. Scores on the checklist may not be sensitive to change. As dementia advances, scores may decrease because certain behaviors may have ceased.

PROCEDURE: There are two parts of the checklist. In the context of the interview, with reference to each one of 26 specific behavior items in turn, the respondent is asked first "if your relative has had any of these problems. If so, how often has this problem occurred during the past week?" Next, if the problem has occurred, the respondent is asked, "How much does the behavior bother or upset you when it happens?" Respondents are given a list of the scaled response choices to facilitate the interview process (Zarit & Zarit, 1990).

SAMPLE ITEMS: "Asks the same question over and over," "Forgets what day it is," and "Becomes angry" (Zarit & Zarit, 1990, p. 6).

SCORING: Frequency responses are scored 0 (*never occurred*), 1 (*has occurred, but not in last week*), 2 (*1 or 2 times in last week*), 3 (*3 to 6 times in last week*), or 4 (*daily or often*). Reaction ratings are scored 0 (*not at all*), 1 (*a little*), 2 (*moderately*), 3 (*very much*), or 4 (*extremely*). The frequency of problems is the sum of scores for frequency items. The difficulty caregivers are having coping with dementia-related problems is the sum of the scores for their reactions. Mean distress scores may also be calculated by dividing the sum of reaction scores by number of behavior problems reported (Zarit & Zarit, 1990). Zarit (1982) found that a cross-product score, calculated by multiplying frequency by reaction, was a predictor of caregiver burden.

SOURCE: The instrument and instructions for its use are available for a small fee from the Gerontology Center at Pennsylvania State University.

REFERENCES

Neundorfer, M. M. (1991). Coping and health outcomes in spouse caregivers of persons with dementia. *Nursing Research, 40,* 260-265.

Teri, L., Truax, P., Logsden, R., Uomoto, J., Vitaliano, P., & Zarit, S. H. (1990). *Assessment of behavioral problems in dementia: The Revised Memory and Behavior Problems Checklist.* Unpublished paper, Department of Psychiatry and Behavioral Sciences, University of Washington Medical Center.

Zarit, J. M. (1982). *Predictors of burden and distress for caregivers of senile dementia patients.* Unpublished doctoral dissertation, University of Southern California.

Zarit, S. H., Anthony, C. R., & Boutselis, M. (1987). Interventions with caregivers of dementia patients: Comparison of two approaches. *Psychology and Aging, 2,* 225-232.

Zarit, S. H., & Zarit, J. M. (1990). *The Memory and Behavior Problems Checklist and the Burden Interview.* (Available from the authors at address listed above)

MINI-MENTAL STATE EXAMINATION (MMSE)

AUTHORS: Marshal F. Folstein, Susan E. Folstein, and
            Paul R. McHugh
ADDRESS: Marshal F. Folstein, MD, Chairman
            Department of Psychiatry
            New England Medical Center #1007
            750 Washington Street
            Boston, MA 02111

DESCRIPTION: The Mini-Mental State Examination (MMSE) is a screening test for cognitive impairment that has been widely used in practice and research. It is an 11-item instrument requiring 5 to 10 minutes to administer. The test concentrates on cognitive aspects of mental functioning but does not address "mood, abnormal mental experiences and the form of thinking" (Folstein, Folstein, & McHugh, 1975, p. 189). Items are designed to screen for orientation, memory, attention, recall, and the ability to name, follow instructions, write a sentence, and copy a polygon. The MMSE was not designed to be used alone as a diagnostic tool.

PSYCHOMETRIC PROPERTIES: The tool has been "found reliable in field studies and hospital settings" (Folstein & Folstein, 1994, p. 224). Test-retest (0.89) and interrater (0.82) reliability have been reported for samples of psychiatric and neurological patients (Anthony, LeResche, Niaz, VonKorff, & Folstein, 1982). MMSE scores of selected samples have correlated well with Wechsler Adult Intelligence Scale (Britton & Savage, 1966) scores and with computerized tomography of the brain. Population norms have been reported by Crum, Anthony, Bassett, and Folstein (1993), who studied a representative U.S. sample selected between 1980 and 1984 ($N = 18,056$). A clinician or researcher can use the tables they generated to compare scores of individuals or samples with national norms for specific age groups while taking age and education into account.

PROCEDURE: Specific instructions are provided in the paper by Folstein et al. (1975). Before administration of the test, the respondent is made comfortable, and rapport is established. During the screening, success is praised, and if the respondent finds particular items difficult, they are not pressed.

SAMPLE ITEMS: "What is the season?" and "Point to a pencil and a watch. Have the patient name them as you point" (Crum et al., 1993, p. 2387).

SCORING: The maximum score is 30. Among persons over 65, 95% have scores of 24 or higher. Scores below 24 occur in delirium, dementia, and severe depression in the elderly and in mental retardation (Folstein & Folstein, 1994, p. 224). Scores of 17 and below are more common among adults with 8 or fewer years of education (Crum et al., 1993, p. 2387).

SOURCE: Copies of the instrument appear in Folstein et al. (1975) and Crum et al. (1993). The MMSE has been translated into several different languages.

REFERENCES

Anthony, J. C., LeResche, L., Niaz, U., VonKorff, M. R., & Folstein, M. F. (1982). Limits of the "Mini-Mental State" as a screening test for dementia and delirium among hospital patients. *Psychological Medicine, 12,* 397-408.

Britton, P. G., & Savage, R. D. (1966). A short form of the WAIS for use with the aged. *British Journal of Psychiatry, 112,* 417-418.

Crum, R. M., Anthony, J. C., Bassett, S. S., & Folstein, M. F. (1993). Population-based norms for the Mini-Mental State Examination by age and education level. *Journal of the American Medical Association, 269,* 2386-2391.

Folstein, M. F., & Folstein, S. E. (1994). Neuropsychiatric assessment of syndromes of altered mental state. In W. R. Hazard, E. L. Bierman, J. P. Blass, W. H. Ettinger, Jr., J. B. Halter, & R. Andres (Eds.), *Principles of geriatric medicine and gerontology* (3rd ed., pp. 221-228). New York: McGraw-Hill.

Folstein, M. F., Folstein, S. E., & McHugh, P. R. (1975). "Mini-Mental State": A practical method for grading the cognitive state of patients for the clinician. *Journal of Psychiatric Research, 12,* 189-195.

MINIMUM DATA SET (MDS) COGNITIVE PERFORMANCE SCALE (CPS)

AUTHORS: John N. Morris, Brant E. Fries, David R. Mehr,
Catherine Hawes, Charles Phillips, Vincent Mor,
and Lewis A. Lipsitz

ADDRESS: Dr. John N. Morris
Hebrew Rehabilitation Center for the Aged
1200 Centre Street
Boston, MA 02131

DESCRIPTION: The Minimum Data Set (MDS) Cognitive Performance Scale (CPS) was designed to be completed with responses to five cognitive items from the MDS. The MDS is the care assessment component of the Resident Assessment Instrument (RAI; Morris et al., 1991) mandated to be completed for all residents in U.S. nursing homes participating in Medicaid or Medicare programs. The CPS was developed to be used by clinicians and investigators to assign residents to one of seven hierarchical cognitive performance categories (Morris et al., 1994, p. M174). The five MDS items used to derive a CPS score, using branching decision rules, relate to whether the resident (a) is comatose or not, (b) has cognitive skills for daily decision making, (c) can be understood by others, (d) has short-term memory allowing recall after 5 minutes, and (e) is dependent or independent in eating (p. M182).

PSYCHOMETRIC PROPERTIES: The authors used two nursing home samples ($N = 284$) to develop a model for deriving a simple scale that could predict Mini-Mental State Examination (MMSE) and Test for Severe Impairment (TSI) scores (see entries in this book). Their goal was "to identify the best system of hierarchical categories that would describe cognitive functional performances" (Morris et al., 1994, p. M176). With the CPS as derived, scores corresponded closely with MMSE and TSI scores (p. M174). Means of MMSE and TSI scores descended across the seven CPS categories. CPS scores and nursing judgments about orientation were compared to show the sensitivity (range 0.86 to 0.95) and specificity (range 0.92 to 0.93) for the CPS (p. M179). To test the model of the proposed CPS, the authors studied CPS distributions for two large national sets of MDS data ($ns = 2,172$ and 6,663). The frequencies for the seven CPS hierarchical categories in the two large samples were comparable. Reliability of MDS ratings had been estimated for independent assessments of residents ($N = 123$) made by licensed nursing personnel in 13 facilities in five states (Hawes et al., 1995, p. 173). The specific MDS items used in the CPS had reliabilities (Spearman-Brown intraclass correlation coefficients) ranging from 0.77 to 1.00 (Morris et al., 1994, p. M177).

PROCEDURE: To derive a CPS score, the clinician or researcher gathers reliable MDS data and applies specified branching decision rules that appear in Morris et al. (1994, p. M178).

SAMPLE ITEM: "Short-Term Memory OK. Intent: To determine ability to recall what was learned or known after 5 minutes. Coding: (0) Memory OK—appears to recall after 5 minutes; (1) Memory Problem" (Morris et al., 1994, p. M182).

SCORING: The seven categories to which residents may be assigned with the CPS Decision Rules are 0 (*intact*), 1 (*borderline intact*), 2 (*mild impairment*), 3 (*moderate impairment*), 4 (*moderately severe impairment*), 5 (*severe impairment*), and 6 (*very severe impairment*).

SOURCE: The CPS is copyrighted by the authors. The MDS items used for the CPS, the decision tree rules used to derive a CPS score, and an example of how to apply the rules appear in Morris et al. (1994).

REFERENCES

Hawes, C., Morris, J. N., Phillips, C., Mor, V., Fries, B. E., & Nonemaker, S. (1995). Reliability estimates for the Minimum Data Set for nursing home resident assessment and care screening. *Gerontologist, 35,* 172-178.

Morris, J. N., Fries, B. E., Mehr, D. R., Hawes, C., Phillips, C., Mor, V., & Lipsitz, L. A. (1994). MDS Cognitive Performance Scale. *Journal of Gerontology: Medical Sciences, 49,* M174-M182.

Morris, J. N., Hawes, C., Murphy, K., Nonemaker, S., Phillips, C. D., Fries, B. E., & Mor, V. (Eds.). (1991). *Resident Assessment Instrument training manual and resource guide.* Natwick, MA: Eliot.

MODIFIED MINI-MENTAL STATE EXAMINATION (3MS)

AUTHORS: Evelyn Lee Teng and Helena Chang Chui
ADDRESS: Evelyn Lee Teng, PhD
            CNH 5641, Department of Neurology
            University of Southern California School of Medicine
            2025 Zonal Avenue
            Los Angeles, CA 90033

DESCRIPTION: The Modified Mini-Mental State (3MS) examination is a brief screening test for cognitive status and dementia, a modification of the classic Mini-Mental State Examination (MMSE; see entry in this book). The modification extends the ranges of scores from 0-30 to 0-100. The 3MS samples a wider range of cognitive abilities; some items on the 3MS have a range of scores where comparable items on the MMSE have only pass or fail options. The changes in this test make it potentially useful in differentiating among nondemented persons and among individuals with advanced dementias. In addition to its clinical uses for screening and assessment (Siu, 1991), the 3MS has been used to measure change in cognitive status in intervention studies (Abraham, Neundorfer, & Currie, 1992) and has potential uses in prospective and epidemiological studies.

PSYCHOMETRIC PROPERTIES: The MMSE, from which the 3MS is derived, is widely used and considered reliable and valid. To establish reliability for the 3MS, MMSE results for 249 patients with various dementias were rescored using 3MS criteria. Agreement between two independent raters for one item (drawing intersecting pentagons), using 3MS criteria, was high. The means and standard deviations were 5.49 ± 3.55 and 5.44 ± 3.57. Scores for this item, which has a potential score of 10, were identical in 80%, differed by 1 point in 16%, and differed by 2 points in 4% of the 249 cases. Pearson's correlation for the sets of scores for the two tests was 0.98 ($p < 0.0001$). Sensitivity of the 3MS is indicated by the analysis of scores for second administrations of the MMSE ($N = 90$). Compared with MMSE scores, the 3MS scores provided better discrimination of cognitive deterioration.

PROCEDURE: The tester makes an effort to make the subject comfortable and to establish a rapport. Generally, successes with the test are praised, and the examiner avoids pressing in areas where the subject has difficulty. The test usually takes about 15 minutes to administer, but there are no time limits. The test has two parts. In the first, the subject responds orally to items that address orientation, memory, and attention. In the second part, abilities to name, follow verbal and written commands, write a sentence, and copy intersecting polygons are tested. Specific recommendations for administration, including some instructions to be followed verbatim, are provided in Teng and Chui (1987). In their article, the authors did not describe procedures and scoring rules that are the same as for the MMSE. Therefore, to complete preparation to administer the 3MS, users need also to read the original Folstein, Folstein, and McHugh (1975) paper on the MMSE.

SAMPLE ITEMS:

> I shall say three words for you to remember. Repeat them after I have said
> *all three* words . . . shirt . . . brown . . . honesty. (Teng & Chui, 1987,
> p. 314)
> What animals have four legs? (p. 315)
> In what way are laughing and crying alike? (p. 315)

SCORING: Specific scoring rules for each item are provided in the article describing instrument development (Teng & Chui, 1987). Scores range between 0 and 100, with 80 or less indicating dementia (Abraham et al., 1992). The 3MS form facilitates calculations of both MMSE and 3MS scores so that comparisons may be made with prior MMSE findings.

SOURCE: The instrument is reprinted in the article describing its development (Teng & Chui, 1987).

REFERENCES

Abraham, I. L., Neundorfer, M. M., & Currie, L. J. (1992). Effects of group interventions on cognition and depression in nursing home residents. *Nursing Research, 41,* 196-202.
Folstein, M. F., Folstein, S. E., & McHugh, P. R. (1975). "Mini-Mental State": A practical method for grading the cognitive state of patients for the clinician. *Journal of Psychiatric Research, 12,* 189-195.
Siu, A. L. (1991). Screening for dementia and investigating its causes. *Annals of Internal Medicine, 115,* 122-132.
Teng, E. L., & Chui, H. C. (1987). The Modified Mini-Mental State (3MS) examination. *Journal of Clinical Psychiatry, 48,* 314-318.

MORSE FALL SCALE

AUTHORS: Janice M. Morse, Robert M. Morse, and Suzanne J. Tylko
ADDRESS: Janice M. Morse, RN, PhD
             International Institute for Qualitative Methodology
             Extension Centre—6th Floor
             University of Alberta
             8303 112th Street
             Edmonton, Alberta T6G 2T4, Canada

DESCRIPTION: The Morse Fall Scale is a quick and simple method to identify patients at risk for falling so that prevention measures can be adopted. The scale, which will classify most, but not all, patients who will fall, consists of six scored items. Morse, Morse, and Tylko (1989) defined falls as events in which the patient came to rest on the floor (p. 367).

PSYCHOMETRIC PROPERTIES: To develop the scale, the investigators examined physiological and environmental variables for 200 patients, 100 who had fallen and 100 randomly selected controls who had not. Using discriminant analysis, they found that six variables classified patients as to whether they had fallen: history of falling, secondary diagnosis, ambulatory aids, IV therapy, gait abnormalities, and mental status. Fall scale weights were calculated for each item variable. Validity for the scale was established by (a) repeating the procedure after randomly splitting the database, (b) examining the cases that had been incorrectly classified as false positives or false negatives, and (c) doing prospective testing in three different types of clinical settings ($N = 2,689$). The scale was sensitive to changes in a patient's condition. Interrater reliability was estimated at 0.96.

PROCEDURE: The scale, which takes less than 3 minutes to complete, can be used as part of the nurse's daily work. The investigators suggest that it not be adopted, however, unless there is a plan in place to protect patients who are found to be at high risk. Use of the scale without emphasis on prevention could lead to increased use of restraints.

ITEMS:

1. History of Falling:	
No	0
Yes	25
2. Secondary Diagnosis:	
No	0
Yes	15
3. Ambulatory Aid:	
None/bedrest/nurse assist	0
Crutches/cane/walker	15
Furniture	30
4. Intravenous Therapy/Heparin Lock:	
No	0
Yes	20
5. Gait:	
Normal/bedrest/wheelchair	0
Weak	10
Impaired	20
6. Mental Status:	
Oriented to own ability	0
Overestimates/forgets limitations	15

(Morse, Morse, & Tylko, 1989, p. 371)

SCORING: Scores are totaled, and the maximum score is 125. Items 1 through 4 are self-explanatory. For some items, however, authors' definitions are needed. *Gait:* With a normal gait, the patient walks with head erect, arms swinging freely at the side and striding unhesitantly. With a weak gait, the patient is stooped but able to lift the head while walking. Support from furniture is sought with a light touch just for reassurance. Steps are short, and the patient may shuffle. When gait is impaired, the patient may have difficulty rising from a chair, the patient's head is down, and poor balance is evident from the patient's grasping of furniture, a person, or a walking aid for support. For those who use wheelchairs, scores are given for performance on transfer to the wheelchair. *Mental Status:* Ask the patient for self-assessment of ambulatory ability: "Do you go to the bathroom alone? Do you need assistance going to the bathroom?" Verify answers by checking ambulation orders. Setting the score for designating high risk is a matter of judgment. Setting the score too low may lead to unnecessarily increasing costs. If the score is too high, potential fallers will not be identified. For their study site, the authors set 16 as the score for high risk.

SOURCE: The scale is reprinted in Morse, Morse, and Tylko (1989). A 12-minute video, *Using the Morse Scale,* is available for a small fee by writing and sending a blank tape to Mr. R. Robinson, Audiovisual Department, Glenrose Rehabilitation Hospital, 10230-111 Avenue, Edmonton, Alberta T5G OB7, Canada.

REFERENCES

Morse, J. M., Black, C., Oberle, K., & Donahue, P. (1989). A prospective study to identify the fall-prone patient. *Social Sciences and Medicine, 28,* 81-86.
Morse, J. M., Morse, R. M., & Tylko, S. J. (1989). Development of a scale to identify the fall-prone patient. *Canadian Journal of Aging, 8,* 366-377.

MULTIDIMENSIONAL OBSERVATION SCALE OF ELDERLY SUBJECTS (MOSES)

AUTHORS: Edward Helmes, Kalman G. Csapo, and Judith-Ann Short
ADDRESS: Dr. Edward Helmes
            St. Mary's Hospital
            35 Grosvenor Street
            London, Ontario N6A 1Y6, Canada

DESCRIPTION: The MOSES is a 40-item observer-rated multidimensional measure of five areas of functioning: self-care, disoriented behavior, depressed/anxious mood, irritable behavior, and withdrawn behavior. There is an eight-item subscale for each of the five areas. The tool was designed to be completed by a member of the nursing staff—including nursing assistants—in daily contact with the resident. The MOSES can be used to plan placement (Sloane & Mathew, 1991), monitor effects of relocation (Bellin, 1990), and evaluate clinical progress or the effects of treatment programs.

PSYCHOMETRIC PROPERTIES: The initial sample for testing the MOSES was 2,542 individuals (70% female), with an average age of 81.3 and an average length of stay of 41.7 months, who resided in 45 diverse long-term care settings in Ontario, Canada. According to Travis (1988), who considered

MOSES "the most complete observer-rated functional assessment tool available" (p. 143), the tool has "strong content validity." Predictive validity was confirmed in comparisons of MOSES scores between patient groups with different discharge outcomes. MOSES scores were significantly correlated with composite scores measuring overall physical disability (N = 2,519). Investigators used Zung's Depression Status Inventory (see entry in this book; N = 32), the Robertson Short Mental Status Questionnaire (Robertson, Rockwood, & Stolee, 1982; N = 33), the London Psychogeriatric Rating Scale (Hersch, Kral, & Palmer, 1978; N = 140), the Kingston Dementia Rating Scale (Lawson, Rodenburg, & Dykes, 1977; N = 24), and a shortened version of the Physical and Mental Impairment-of-Function Evaluation (Gurel, Linn, & Linn, 1972; PAMIE; N = 230) to confirm convergent and discriminant validity. Interrater reliabilities using intraclass correlations ranged between 0.58 (depression) and 0.97 (self-care). Internal consistency, measured with the alpha coefficient, ranged from 0.78 (withdrawal) to 0.87 (disorientation). Pruchno, Kleban, and Resch (1988) conducted a psychometric assessment of MOSES. See their article for the suggestion about a 24-item revision of the MOSES.

PROCEDURE: A staff member in daily contact with the older person completes the tool by circling explicit response options for each of the 40 items. The subject need not cooperate with the assessment; therefore, the measure is unobtrusive.

SAMPLE ITEM: Physical Mobility.

> On most days in the past week, when getting around inside the building, the resident:
>
> 1. Walked without any assistance
> 2. Moved independently with mechanical assistance (for example, walked alone with a cane or walker or crutches, or propelled himself in a wheelchair)
> 3. Walked with the physical assistance of staff
> 4. Remained bedfast or chairfast (*chairfast* refers to residents who were moved from bed to a chair during the daytime, but otherwise were quite immobile) (Helmes, Csapo, & Short, 1987, p. 401)

SCORING: Raters choose the alternative that best describes behavior "during the daytime in the past week." Items are rated on a 4- or 5-point Likert scale, with lower scores associated with higher levels of function. See Pruchno et al. (1988) for suggested revisions of the original scoring procedures.

SOURCE: The instrument is included in the article describing its development (Helmes et al., 1987).

REFERENCES

Bellin, C. (1990). Relocating adult day care: Its impact on persons with dementia. *Journal of Gerontological Nursing, 16*(3), 11-14.

Gurel, L., Linn, M. W., & Linn, B. S. (1972). Physical and mental impairment-of-function evaluation in the aged: The PAMIE scale. *Journal of Gerontology, 27,* 83-90.

Helmes, E., Csapo, K. G., & Short, J.-A. (1987). Standardization and validation of the Multidimensional Observation Scale for Elderly Subjects (MOSES). *Journal of Gerontology, 42,* 395-405.

Hersch, E. L., Kral, V. A., & Palmer, R. B. (1978). Clinical value of the London Psychogeriatric Rating Scale. *Journal of the American Geriatrics Society, 26,* 348-354.

Lawson, J. S., Rodenburg, M., & Dykes, J. A. (1977). A dementia rating scale for use with psychogeriatric patients. *Journal of Gerontology, 32,* 153-159.

Pruchno, R. A., Kleban, M. H., & Resch, N. L. (1988). Psychometric assessment of the multidimensional observation scale for elderly subjects (MOSES). *Journal of Gerontology: Psychological Sciences, 43,* P164-P169.

Robertson, D., Rockwood, K., & Stolee, P. (1982). A short mental status questionnaire. *Canadian Journal of Aging, 1,* 16-20.

Sloane, P. D., & Mathew, L. J. (1991). An assessment and care planning strategy for nursing home residents with dementia. *Gerontologist, 31,* 128-131.

Travis, S. S. (1988). Observer-rated functional assessments for institutionalized elders. *Nursing Research, 37,* 138-143.

NEECHAM CONFUSION SCALE (NEECHAM)

AUTHORS: Virginia J. Neelon, M. T. Champagne, and
            E. S. McConnell
ADDRESS: Virginia J. Neelon, RN, PhD
            School of Nursing
            CB#7460, Carrington Hall
            University of North Carolina at Chapel Hill
            Chapel Hill, NC 27599

DESCRIPTION: The purpose of the Neecham Confusion Scale (Neecham) is to monitor and predict acute confusion. The scale "permits rapid bedside documentation of: 1) normal information processing; 2) early subtle cues preceding acute confusion behavior; and 3) acute confusion" (Champagne, Neelon, McConnell, & Funk, 1987, p. 4A). Assessments to complete the Neecham are made by an observer who uses a relatively unobtrusive method. There are nine scaled items in three subscales for (a) cognitive processing, (b) behavior, and (c) physiological control. Subscale items have criteria describing observations typical of particular levels of confusion. Measurement of vital signs and ratings for incontinence and oxygen saturation are also included. The scale is reported to be sensitive to early onset of confusion (Neelon, Funk, Carlson, & Champagne, 1989, p. 65A). Smith, Breitbart, and Platt (1995) suggested that the Neecham could be used for long-term longitudinal and follow-up studies (p. 69) and for screening in large, varied populations "as long as the physical parameters could be easily obtained" (p. 67).

PSYCHOMETRIC PROPERTIES: Reliability was demonstrated with data from repeated measures of 35 hospital and nursing home patients: internal consistency (alpha = 0.86), interrater reliability (0.96), and test-retest reliability (0.98). Neecham scores were correlated (0.81) with scores on the Mini-Mental State Examination (MMSE; see entry in this book; Champagne et al., 1987, p. 4A). Neelon et al. (1989) evaluated 158 medical patients aged 64 and over and found that Neecham scores at 24 and below "predicted confusion with a sensitivity of 0.95 and a specificity of 0.78" (p. 65A). The patients were also rated with three "key clinical indicators" for development of acute confusion: (a) the criteria of the third edition of the *Diagnostic and Statistical Manual of Mental Disorders* (American Psychiatric Association, 1980), (b) the MMSE, and (c) report of a mental status problem documented in the clinical record. Scores on the Neecham for "normal," "early change," and "moderate to severe" groups were significantly related to number of clinical indicators (Neelon et al., 1989, p. 65A).

PROCEDURE: Ratings are assigned based on observations made during a specific clinical interaction. Many of the Neecham assessments draw on data routinely gathered by nurses.

SAMPLE ITEM: Behavior-Appearance:

2	*Controls posture, maintains appearance, hygiene:* appropriately gowned or dressed, personally tidy, clean. Posture in bed/chair normal.
1	*Either posture or appearance disturbed:* some disarray of clothing/bed or personal appearance, or some loss of control of posture, position.
0	*Both posture and appearance abnormal:* disarrayed, poor hygiene, unable to maintain posture in bed.

(Neelon, Champagne, & McConnell, 1985)

SCORING: The range of scores for the Neecham is 0 to 30. The authors have used the following cutoff scores: scores above 24 for not confused, 24 to 20 for mild or early development of confusion, and 20 to 0 for moderate to severe confusion (Neelon, Champagne, McConnell, Carlson, & Funk, 1992, p. 281).

SOURCE: Copies of the instrument and an instruction guide for administering and scoring the Neecham are available from the authors. They hold a copyright.

REFERENCES

American Psychiatric Association. (1980). *Diagnostic and statistical manual of mental disorders* (3rd ed.). Washington, DC: Author.

Champagne, M. T., Neelon, V. J., McConnell, E. S., & Funk, S. (1987). The Neecham Confusion Scale: Assessing acute confusion. *Gerontologist, 27,* 4A.

Neelon, V. J., Champagne, M. T., & McConnell, E. S. (1985). *Neecham Confusion Scale.* (Available from the authors at address listed above)

Neelon, V. J., Champagne, M. T., McConnell, E. S., Carlson, J. R., & Funk, S. G. (1992). Use of the Neecham Confusion Scale to assess acute confusional states of hospitalized older patients. In S. Funk, E. Tournquist, M. Champagne, & R. Wiese (Eds.), *Key aspects of eldercare: Managing falls, incontinence, and cognitive impairment* (pp. 278-289). New York: Springer.

Neelon, V. J., Funk, S. G., Carlson, J. R., & Champagne, M. T. (1989). The Neecham Confusion Scale. *Gerontologist, 29,* 65A.

Smith, M. J., Breitbart, W. S., & Platt, M. M. (1995). A critique of instruments and methods to detect, diagnose, and rate delirium. *Journal of Pain and Symptom Management, 10*(1), 35-77.

NURSES' OBSERVATION SCALE FOR GERIATRIC PATIENTS (NOSGER)

AUTHOR: René Spiegel
ADDRESS: Professor Dr. René Spiegel
            Dementia Project Unit
            Sandoz Pharma Ltd.
            CH-4002 Basel, Switzerland

DESCRIPTION: The NOSGER is intended for use with psychogeriatric inpatients and outpatients. It contains 30 items, each describing an everyday behavior that can be rated by a caregiver. Ratings are for frequency of behaviors, within the 2 weeks before evaluation, on a 5-point scale. The scale is used to assess six dimensions of behavior typical in psychogeriatric patients: disturbances of memory, disturbances of instrumental activities of daily living (IADLs), disturbances of activities of daily living (ADLs), depressed mood, impaired social behavior, and disturbing behavior. Scale items were derived from two previously published instruments: the GERRI (Schwartz, 1983) and the NOSIE (Honigfeld, 1974).

PSYCHOMETRIC PROPERTIES: The variables and dimensions for the instrument are defined behaviorally. The developers conducted three independent validation studies. The first was with three groups, each with 20 participants, of elderly persons living in the community or in institutions in or near Basel, Switzerland; a German version of the tool was administered. Later, in Canada, 55 patients with primary degenerative dementia of the Alzheimer's type (PDD-AT; $n = 27$ in community and $n = 28$ in institutions) were studied with the instrument. The third study was carried out with PDD-AT patients living in the community or in institutions who were participants in a "multicenter drug trial" in 33 centers in 11 countries. Concurrent validity was demonstrated through high correlations with other instruments thought to assess similar relevant areas. Spearman rank correlations ranged between 0.68 and 0.93 for test-retest reliability and between 0.60 and 0.91 for interrater reliability, all significant at the 0.001 level. The dimension scores of the NOSGER are differentially sensitive to change over time, and sensitivity in two dimensions (memory and IADLs) is similar to the sensitivity of the Mini-Mental State Examination (see entry in this book;

Tremmel & Spiegel, 1993). Changes in the six NOSGER dimensions corre-lated with ratings of treatment efficacy made independently by physicians.

PROCEDURE: The rater receives brief oral instructions duplicated in print on the scale. Raters are advised to review all items before administration, but training of raters is not necessary.

SAMPLE ITEMS: "Shaves or puts on make-up, combs hair without help" and "Follows favorite radio or TV programs" (Spiegel et al., 1991, p. 346).

SCORING: Items are scored from 1 (*all the time*) to 5 (*none of the time*). Some items are scored in reverse. Low scores represent little or no distur-bance, and high scores reflect severe dysfunction. Tentative normative data suggest that cutoff scores are 10 for ADLs, and 15 for both memory and IADL dimensions (Tremmel & Spiegel, 1993).

SOURCE: The instrument is available from the author free of charge in English, French, German, and a number of other European languages. A reprint of the tool appears in Spiegel et al. (1991).

REFERENCES

Honigfeld, G. (1974). NOSIE-3O: History and current status of its use in pharmacopsychia-tric research. In P. Pichot (Ed.), *Modern problems of pharmacopsychiatry: Vol. 7. Psychological measurement in psycho-pharmacology* (pp. 238-263). Basel, Switzerland: Karger.

Schwartz, G. E. (1983). Development and validation of geriatric evaluation by relatives rating instrument (GERRI). *Psychological Reports, 53,* 479-488.

Spiegel, R., Brunner, C., Ermini-Funfschilling, D., Monsch, A., Notter, M., Puxty, J., & Tremmel, L. (1991). A new behavioral assessment scale for geriatric out- and in-patients: The NOSGER (Nurses' Observation Scale for Geriatric Patients). *Journal of the American Geriatric Society, 39,* 339-347.

Tremmel, L., & Spiegel, R. (1993). Clinical experience with the NOSGER (Nurses' Obser-vation Scale for Geriatric Patients): Tentative normative data and sensitivity to change. *International Journal of Geriatric Psychiatry, 8,* 311-317.

NURSING HOME BEHAVIOR PROBLEM
SCALE (NHBPS)

AUTHORS: Wayne A. Ray, Jo A. Taylor, Michael J. Lichtenstein,
             and Keith G. Meador

ADDRESS: Wayne A. Ray, PhD
             Department of Preventive Medicine
             Vanderbilt University School of Medicine
             Nashville, TN 37232

DESCRIPTION: The Nursing Home Behavior Problem Scale (NHBPS) was developed "to measure the specific behavior problems that in the nursing home setting are so disruptive or stressful as to lead to use of antipsychotic drugs or physical restraints" (Ray, Taylor, Lichtenstein, & Meador, 1992, p. M10). It is a 29-item scale designed to be completed by nurses, nursing assistants, or other caregivers.

PSYCHOMETRIC PROPERTIES: Data for validation studies were gathered for 564 residents of six nursing homes. Interrater reliability (Pearson r) for pairs of raters ranged from 0.69 to 0.92. For a subsample ($n = 122$), correlations between NHBPS scores and scores on two similar instruments were 0.75 (Nurse-Oriented Scale for Inpatient Evaluation; Honigfeld, 1974) and 0.91 (Cohen-Mansfield Agitation Inventory; see entry in this book). Average scores for residents who were receiving psychoactive drugs, had been physically restrained, or were considered impaired were higher (21.2) than scores for residents not receiving drugs and not restrained (10.0; Ray et al., 1992, p. M13). Cluster analyses revealed six subscales: (a) uncooperative or aggressive behaviors, (b) irrational or restless behaviors, (c) sleep problems, (d) annoying behaviors, (e) inappropriate behaviors, and (f) dangerous behaviors (p. M12).

PROCEDURE: A respondent who is familiar with the resident rates each behavior for frequency of occurrence during the last 3 days (0 = *never,* 1 = *sometimes,* 2 = *often,* 3 = *usually,* 4 = *always*). Completion of the scale requires from 3 to 5 minutes. The investigators observed that ratings assigned by nursing assistants were "generally lower and less variable" (Ray et al., 1992, p. M11) than those made by nurses. Among nurse/nurse assistant pairs of raters, there were some instances of large differences between ratings. The authors suggest that reliability of scores may be improved by training raters or by using more quantitative language to distinguish frequencies (p. M13).

SAMPLE ITEMS: "Argues, threatens or curses," "Talks, mutters, or mumbles to herself," and "Disturbs others during the night" (Ray et al., 1992, pp. M15-M16).

SCORING: The rater circles the number corresponding to a frequency for each of the behaviors on the scale. NHBPS scores are the sum of item ratings. The range of scores is between 0 and 116.

SOURCE: A copy of the scale is in the appendix to Ray et al. (1992).

REFERENCES

Honigfeld, G. (1974). NOSIE-30: History and current status of its use in pharmacopsychiatric research. *Modern Problems in Pharmacopsychiatry, 7,* 238-263.

Ray, W. A., Taylor, J. A., Lichtenstein, M. J., & Meador, K. G. (1992). The Nursing Home Behavior Problem Scale. *Journal of Gerontology: Medical Sciences, 47,* M9-M16.

NUTRITIONAL RISK INDEX (NRI)

AUTHORS: Frederic D. Wolinsky, Rodney M. Coe,
            William Alex McIntosh, Karen S. Kubena,
            John M. Prendergast, M. Noel Chavez,
            Douglas K. Miller, James C. Romeis, and
            Wendall A. Landmann

ADDRESS: Frederic D. Wolinsky, PhD, Professor of Medicine
            Indiana University, Department of Medicine
            Regenstreif Institute, RHC/5th
            1001 West Tenth Street
            Indianapolis, IN 46202-2859

DESCRIPTION: The Nutritional Risk Index (NRI) was developed specifically to screen elderly persons for "risk of developing nutritionally related disabilities" (Wolinsky et al., 1990, p. 1549). The NRI "taps five important dimensions of nutritional risk, including mechanics of food intake, prescribed dietary restrictions, morbid conditions affecting food intake, discomfort associated with the outcomes of food intake, and significant changes in dietary habits" (p. 1549).

PSYCHOMETRIC PROPERTIES: NRI items were derived, in part, from the U.S. government's National Health and Nutrition Examination Survey (Department of Health, Education, and Welfare, 1977). The instrument was tested initially with a random sample ($N = 401$) in the St. Louis area (Wolinsky, Coe, Chavez, Prendergast, & Miller, 1986). Alpha coefficients ranged from 0.54 to 0.60, and test-retest correlations ranged between 0.65 and 0.71. Factor analysis confirmed an expected five-factor structure that accounted for 47.9% of the variance (Wolinsky et al., 1986, pp. 984-985). Predictive validity was supported when regression models for forecasting use of health services by the elderly were enhanced with the addition of NRI scores (Wolinsky et al., 1990, p. 1551). Scores on the NRI were correlated with other measures of nutritional status, such as body mass index (p. 1552). Further support for validity of the tool was demonstrated with comparisons between respondents, divided into high- and low-risk groups on the basis of NRI scores. The highs were more likely to be rated "emaciated" and had more physician and emergency room visits and more hospitalizations (p. 1551). The St. Louis findings were confirmed in several other studies.

PROCEDURE: The NRI is suitable for pencil-and-paper completion or for use in a face-to-face or telephone interview. The respondent simply answers "yes" or "no" to each of the 16 items.

SAMPLE ITEMS: "Do you now have an illness or condition that interferes with your eating?" and "Do you wear dentures?" (Wolinsky et al., 1990, p. 1550).

SCORING: The score is the number of "yes" responses to the index. A person who scores 8 or more on the NRI is considered at high risk for having "poor nutritional status, poor health status in general, and greater health services utilization levels" (Wolinsky et al., 1990, p. 1553).

SOURCE: The instrument is available from the author. The specific items and their order of administration are available in Wolinsky et al. (1986, 1990).

REFERENCES

Department of Health, Education and Welfare. (1977). Plan and operation of the Health Examination Survey, United States, 1971-1973. USPHS Publication No. (HRA) 77-1310.

Wolinsky, F. D., Coe, R. M., Chavez, M. N., Prendergast, J. M., & Miller, D. K. (1986). Further assessment of the reliability and validity of a nutritional risk index: Analysis of a three-wave panel study of elderly adults. *Health Services Research, 20,* 987-990.

Wolinsky, F. D., Coe, R. M., McIntosh, A., Kubena, K. S., Prendergast, J. M., Chavez, M. N., Miller, D. K., Romeis, J. C., & Landmann, W. A. (1990). Progress in the development of a nutritional risk index. *Journal of Nutrition, 120,* 1549-1553.

PERCEIVED STRESS QUESTIONNAIRE (PSQ)

AUTHORS: Susan Levenstein, Cosimo Prantera, Vilma Varvo, Maria
Lia Scribano, Eva Berto, Arnaldo Andreoli, and Carlo Luzi

ADDRESS: Susan Levenstein, MD
Via Cesare Balbo 43
00184 Rome, Italy

DESCRIPTION: The Perceived Stress Questionnaire (PSQ) is a 30-item instrument designed for use in psychosomatic research. Items elicit, not a list of worries, but the extent to which respondents ("usually," "often," "sometimes," or "almost never") feel "under pressure from them" (Levenstein et al., 1993, p. 29). There are two PSQ forms: Recent (PSQ-R) asks about "last month," and General (PSQ-G) covers the "last year or two."

PSYCHOMETRIC PROPERTIES: Items for the PSQ were selected to be diversely applicable, yet "interpretable as specific to a variety of real-life situations" (Levenstein et al., 1993, p. 20). They reflect "psychosocial factors thought to precipitate relapses" (p. 20) among persons with ulcerative colitis, duodenal ulcer, and asthma. Both forms of the PSQ are internally consistent; the alpha coefficient for PSQ-G was 0.90, and the alpha for PSQ-R was 0.92. A correlation for test-retest reliability ($N = 101$) at approximately 1 week (0.82) demonstrated that the instrument was stable over time; it was also "sensitive to temporal fluctuations in the stress experience" (p. 30). Construct validity was supported by comparing PSQ scores ($N = 230$) with scores on five other measures of stress. Both PSQ-G and PSQ-R scores "were highly correlated with minor physical symptomatology in basically healthy individuals" (p. 26). A principal components factor analysis ($N = 230$) yielded seven factors. In a double-blind study of middle-aged ulcerative colitis patients, the authors found that PSQ-G scores of 46 asymptomatic patients were significantly higher in the "11 with mucosal abnormalities than in the 35 with a normal rectal mucosa" (Levenstein et al., 1994, p. 1219).

PROCEDURE: The tool is phrased in simple language and takes a few minutes to complete. Respondents circle the appropriate choice for each item on the scale.

SAMPLE ITEMS: "Your problems seem to be piling up," "You feel safe and protected," "You have many worries," and "You have trouble relaxing" (Levenstein et al., 1993, p. 32).

SCORING: Eight items are designed to be scored in reverse. General and recent scores can be compared. An overall PSQ index may be calculated, as well as a score for each of the seven subscales.

SOURCE: The instrument and instructions about scoring are available from Dr. Levenstein, who holds the copyright. The PSQ is reprinted in the appendix to Levenstein et al. (1993).

REFERENCES

Levenstein, S., Prantera, C., Varvo, V., Scribano, M. L., Berto, E., Andreoli, A., & Luzi, C. (1994). Psychological stress and disease activity in ulcerative colitis: A multidimensional cross-sectional study. *American Journal of Gastroenterology, 89,* 1219-1225.

Levenstein, S., Prantera, C., Varvo, V., Scribano, M. L., Berto, E., Luzi, C., & Andreoli, A. (1993). Development of the Perceived Stress Questionnaire: A new tool for psychosomatic research. *Journal of Psychosomatic Research, 37*(1), 19-32.

PERCEIVED STRESS SCALE (PSS)

AUTHORS: Sheldon Cohen, Tom Kamarck, and Robin Mermelstein

ADDRESS: Dr. Sheldon Cohen
            Department of Psychology
            Carnegie-Mellon University
            Pittsburgh, PA 15213

DESCRIPTION: The Perceived Stress Scale (PSS) is a 14-item instrument designed to "tap the degree to which respondents find their lives unpredictable, uncontrollable, and overloading: three items central to stress" (Cohen, 1986, p. 717). Items on the scale, which was designed for the general population, "represent situations where persons perceive that their demands exceed their ability to cope" (p. 717). The PSS provides for assessment of nonspecific appraised stress; it does not inquire about particular events or situations.

PSYCHOMETRIC PROPERTIES: The scale is based theoretically on the idea that "the impact of 'objectively' stressful events is, to some degree, determined by one's perception of their stressfulness" (Cohen, Kamarck, & Mermelstein, 1983, p. 385). The PSS was intended for persons with a junior high school education and was originally standardized with college students and individuals participating in a stop-smoking program. PSS scores were correlated, as predicted, "with a range of self-report and behavioral criteria" and were better predictors of health and health-related outcomes than either of two life events scales (p. 393). Internal consistency reliability with college student samples ranged between 0.84 and 0.86. For stop-smoking samples, test-retest reliabilities ($N = 82$) were 0.85 at 2 days and dropped to 0.55 when measured ($N = 64$) at 6-week intervals (p. 390). Cohen and Williamson (1988) studied PSS scores of a large sample ($N = 2,387$) surveyed in a Harris Poll conducted by telephone. The alpha coefficient was 0.75. Grant, Skinkle, and Lipps (1992) studied relocation of a nursing home sample using the PSS. Their "interviewable" residents "understood the items and felt they were relevant to their experience" (p. 838). The alpha coefficient for scores of 69 residents was 0.75 (p. 838). In a longitudinal study of Alzheimer's disease patients ($N = 35$) and their spouse caregivers, Gallagher-Thompson, Brooks, Bliwise, Leader, and Yesavage (1992) found that caregivers' perceived stress was related "both to patients' sundowning behaviors and their subsequent rate of cognitive decline" (p. 810).

PROCEDURE: PSS items ask about frequency of "feelings and thoughts" during the last month. The scale can be administered in writing, orally, or by telephone. Completion usually takes just a few minutes. Ten- and four-item versions of the PSS have also been validated. The 10-item version, shown to be "at least as good a measure of perceived stress as the longer 14-item version" (Cohen & Williamson, 1988, p. 47), includes Items 1 to 3, 6 to 11, and 14. The four-item version includes Items 2, 6, 7, and 14 (p. 34). The four-item version is recommended if the PSS is used in telephone surveys.

SAMPLE ITEM:

In the last month, how often have you been upset because of something that happened unexpectedly?

(0 = *never,* 1 = *almost never,* 2 = *sometimes,* 3 = *fairly often,* 4 = *very often*)
(Cohen et al., 1983, p. 394).

SCORING: Each item has the same five possible responses. Seven items are phrased positively and are therefore scored in reverse (0 = 4, 1 = 3, 2 = 2, 3 = 1, 4 = 0). Higher scores indicate more stress. The range of possible scores for the 14-item scale is 0 to 56. The range of PSS scores for a national probability sample (N = 2,387) was 0 to 45. The mean for scores of both males and females in that sample was 19.62, with a standard deviation of 7.49. The mean for scores of females (M = 20.2; SD = 7.8) was significantly higher than it was for males (M = 18.8; SD = 6.9). The mean score for persons over 65 (n = 296) was 18.5, with a standard deviation of 7.8 (Cohen & Williamson, 1988, p. 48).

SOURCE: The 14-item version of the PSS is reprinted in the appendix to Cohen et al. (1983) and in Cohen and Williamson (1988). It is also available from Dr. Cohen.

REFERENCES

Cohen, S. (1986). Contrasting the Hassles Scale and the Perceived Stress Scale. *American Psychologist, 41,* 716-718.

Cohen, S., Kamarck, T., & Mermelstein, R. (1983). A global measure of perceived stress. *Journal of Health and Social Behavior, 24,* 385-396.

Cohen, S., & Williamson, G. M. (1988). Perceived stress in a probability sample of the United States. In S. Spacapan & S. Oskamp (Eds.), *The social psychology of health* (pp. 31-67). Newbury Park, CA: Sage.

Gallagher-Thompson, D., Brooks, J. O., Bliwise, D., Leader, J., & Yesavage, J. D. (1992). The relations among caregiver stress, "sundowning" symptoms, and cognitive decline in Alzheimer's disease. *Journal of the American Geriatrics Society, 40,* 807-810.

Grant, P. R., Skinkle, R. R., & Lipps, G. (1992). The impact of an institutional relocation on nursing home residents requiring a high level of care. *Gerontologist, 32,* 834-842.

PERFORMANCE ACTIVITIES OF DAILY LIVING (PADL)

AUTHORS: J. B. Kuriansky and Barry J. Gurland
ADDRESS: Dr. Jeanne A. Teresi
            Research Division
            The Hebrew Home for the Aged at Riverdale
            5901 Palisade Avenue
            Riverdale, NY 10471

DESCRIPTION: The Performance Activities of Daily Living (PADL) is a timed test of the performance of selected activities of daily living. It is part of the Comprehensive Assessment and Referral Evaluation (CARE; Gurland et al., 1977-1978), a multidimensional assessment instrument; it may also be used independently. The instrument was designed "to objectively measure the self-care capacity of geriatric psychiatric patients" (Kuriansky & Gurland, 1976, p. 343). There are two versions of the PADL. The original version measures 16 activities of daily living related to eating and drinking, grooming, dressing, bathing, care of the mouth and dentures, communicating, telling time, and walking (p. 346). The examiner uses a variety of commonly available objects as props. A shorter form includes performance tests for drinking, simulated eating, combing hair, and dressing the upper and lower body (Hebrew Home, 1994). In each of the activities of daily living (ADL) areas, the subject is asked to complete the task, and the observer times the performance and rates from two to five sequential behaviors for each ADL area.

PSYCHOMETRIC PROPERTIES: After pretesting showed that "reliability based on independent ratings of the interviewer and the observer was good (i.e., 0.902)" (Kuriansky & Gurland, 1976, p. 348), the original version of the PADL was administered to samples of persons admitted consecutively to psychiatric wards of public hospitals in New York and London ($N = 96$). Each person was seen within 1 week of admission and on two follow-up occasions. Performance on the PADL "was correlated to physical health, mental status and location at follow-up" (p. 349). Validity of the instrument was supported by findings that the "higher the level of independence as measured by the PADL, the better was the patient's health status on medical examination, and the better were his chances for survival and discharge from hospital" (p. 349). Improvement and decline in performance were associated with favorable and unfavorable outcomes, respectively. The objective testing performed with the PADL was more valid than self-reports or reports by informants (p. 349).

PROCEDURE: Before testing is begun, the observer verifies with a responsible person that there are no contraindications for the subject's performance of tasks. The PADL "was designed so that the patient need only get one simple message that he is to demonstrate certain activities" (Kuriansky & Gurland, 1976, p. 347). The instruction to the subject is given once and may be repeated twice. Verbal prompting given after the subject has begun the task affects scoring. If there is no response after 2 minutes, the observer moves on to the next task. Each subtask is completed and scored sequentially.

SAMPLE ITEM: Eating.

> Place foam ball on spoon; place spoon on table in front of participant and say, "Pretend this is food you would eat from a spoon. Show me how you would eat it." Score for the following: a) grasps spoon by handle, b) keeps foam balanced on spoon, c) aims at mouth, and d) touches spoon to mouth. (Kuriansky & Gurland, 1994, p. 2)

SCORING: For the original version, the PADL was scored for the proportion of tested functions performed correctly. A person was "independent" when all tasks were completed without help, "moderately dependent" when his or her score was between 75% and 99%, and "dependent" when his or her score was less than 75%. For the short form, an item is scored 2 if performed without cues, 1 if performed with cues, and 0 if the task is attempted but the subject is unable to do it. Scores for no response, refusal, or not done due to perceptual and/or physical impairment may also be coded.

SOURCE: The original version of the instrument is available from Dr. Barry Gurland. The shorter version (Kuriansky & Gurland, 1994) and its manual (Hebrew Home, 1994) may be obtained from Dr. Jeanne A. Teresi, Research Division, The Hebrew Home for the Aged at Riverdale, 5901 Palisade Avenue, Riverdale, NY 10471.

REFERENCES

Gurland, B. J., Kuriansky, J. B., Sharpe, L. K., Simon, R., Stiller, P., & Birkett, P. (1977-1978). The Comprehensive Assessment and Referral Evaluation (CARE): Rationale, development and reliability. *International Journal of Aging and Human Development, 8,* 9-42.

Hebrew Home for the Aged at Riverdale. (1994). *Performance Activities of Daily Living (PADL) manual.* (Available from Dr. Jeanne A. Teresi, Research Division, The Hebrew Home for the Aged at Riverdale, 5901 Palisade Avenue, Riverdale, NY 10471)

Kuriansky, J. B., & Gurland, B. (1976). Performance test of activities of daily living. *International Journal of Aging and Human Development, 7,* 343-352.

Kuriansky, J. B., & Gurland, B. (1994). *Performance Activities of Daily Living.* (Available from the authors at address listed above)

PHILADELPHIA GERIATRIC CENTER MORALE SCALE REVISED (PGCMS)

AUTHOR: M. Powell Lawton
ADDRESS: M. Powell Lawton
            Philadelphia Geriatric Center
            5301 Old York Road
            Philadelphia, PA 19141

DESCRIPTION: Lawton and his staff developed the Philadelphia Geriatric Center Morale Scale Revised (PGCMS), a measure of subjective well-being, especially for relatively less competent older persons (Lawton, n.d., p. 1). This multidimensional instrument has been widely used to assess the psychological states of older persons. The author's current version of the scale has 17 items. Other investigators (Liang & Bollen, 1985; McCulloch, 1991) have recommended 15-item formats. Lawton noted that the scores on the PGCMS should not be taken as "absolute"; rather, they should be used "in the clinical setting as one assist in helping older persons and their families make decisions" (Lawton, n.d., p. 2). Lawton suggested that a major strength of the instrument is its ability to facilitate dialogue between the respondent and a clinician (p. 3).

PSYCHOMETRIC PROPERTIES: For the original 22-item version of the PGCMS, Lawton (1972) studied responses from residents of homes and housing for the aged and reported split-half (0.74) and test-retest (0.75 to 0.91) reliability. The coefficient for internal consistency was 0.81. PGCMS scores were validated by comparing them with ratings for adjustment made by staff members. In 1975, Lawton reported factor-analytic studies with samples ($N = 828$) of residents of public and limited-income housing in the eastern and midwestern United States. Three "stable and replicable factors" of the PGCMS emerged: Agitation (6 items), Attitude Toward Aging (5 items), and Lonely Dissatisfaction (6 items). Alpha coefficients for these factors were 0.85, 0.81, and 0.85 respectively (p. 87). According to the author, the items grouped together as the Agitation factor "might be used as an old person's manifest anxiety scale" (p. 88). Ryden (1984), who showed that "a sense of control is a significant predictor of morale in institutionalized elderly" (p. 136), reported mean PGCMS scores for skilled and intermediate care samples ($n = 54$; $n = 59$) as 10.77 and 11.24 respectively (p. 132).

PROCEDURE: Lawton recommended that the scale be administered orally, with care not to explain or elaborate items, but merely to repeat them if the respondent has not understood the interviewer. The introduction suggested is "I would like to ask you a few questions. You can just answer yes or no to most of them" (Lawton, n.d., p. 2). For the three items for which there are other responses, the choices are read to the respondent. Depending on the capability of respondents, a pencil-and-paper format could also be used.

SAMPLE ITEMS: "Do little things bother you more this year?" "Are you as happy now as you were when you were younger?" and "Do you have a lot to be sad about?" (Lawton, n.d., p. 4).

SCORING: Responses indicating high morale are scored 1. The sum of these scores is the PGCMS score. Morale scores between 13 and 17 are high, scores between 10 and 12 are midrange, and scores of 9 and below are low (Lawton, n.d., p. 2).

SOURCE: A copy of the PGCMS and its administration and scoring instructions (Lawton, n.d.) are available from the author.

REFERENCES

Lawton, M. P. (1972). The dimensions of morale. In D. Kent, R. Kastenbaum, & S. Sherwood (Eds.), *Research, planning and action for the elderly* (pp. 144-165). New York: Behavioral Publications.

Lawton, M. P. (1975). The Philadelphia Geriatric Center Morale Scale: A revision. *Journal of Gerontology, 30,* 85-88.

Lawton, M. P. (n.d.). *The Philadelphia Geriatric Center Morale Scale: Administration and scoring instructions.* (Available from the author at address listed above)

Liang, J., & Bollen, K. A. (1985). Gender differences in the structure of the Philadelphia Geriatric Center Morale Scale. *Journal of Gerontology, 40,* 468-477.

McCulloch, B. J. (1991). A longitudinal investigation of the factor structure of well-being: The case of the Philadelphia Geriatric Center Morale Scale. *Journal of Gerontology: Psychological Sciences, 46,* P251-P258.

Ryden, M. B. (1984). Morale and perceived control in institutionalized elderly. *Nursing Research, 33,* 130-136.

PITTSBURGH SLEEP QUALITY INDEX (PSQI)

AUTHORS: Daniel J. Buysse, Charles F. Reynolds III,
            Timothy H. Monk, Susan R. Berman, and
            David J. Kupfer
ADDRESS: Daniel J. Buysse, MD
            University of Pittsburgh Medical Center
            Western Psychiatric Institute and Clinic
            3811 O'Hara Street
            Pittsburgh, PA 15213

DESCRIPTION: The Pittsburgh Sleep Quality Index (PSQI) is a 19-item questionnaire designed to measure self-rated sleep patterns in a preceding month. The index yields a global PSQI score and component scores for sleep quality, sleep latency, duration and efficiency of sleep, disturbances of sleep, use of sleep medication, and dysfunction during daytime hours. The 1-month time period in which responses are framed provides information about frequency and/or duration of sleep problems (Buysse, Reynolds, Monk, Berman, & Kupfer, 1989, p. 195). Subjective sleep quality has been found to deteriorate with age. Older subjects have higher PSQI global scores and more variability in scores (Buysse et al., 1991).

PSYCHOMETRIC PROPERTIES: To assess validity, the investigators studied three groups, known to be "normal," "depressed," and "poor sleepers." Items and total scores were stable over time. Alpha coefficient was 0.83 (Buysse et al., 1989, p. 197). PSQI global and component scores distinguished between known groups. A post hoc global PSQI cutoff score of 5 "correctly identified 88.5% (131/148) of all patients and controls (kappa = 0.75, $p < 0.001$). This represents a sensitivity of 89.6% and a specificity of 86.5%" (p. 199). Validity for the PSQI was also supported by some categories of concurrent polysomnographic findings (p. 199).

PROCEDURE: The instrument form is headed by instructions to the respondent. The PSQI was reported to have been "easy to use" for community-dwelling samples. It could be used by a subject independently or completed in an interview.

SAMPLE ITEMS: "During the past month, when have you usually gone to bed at night?" and "During the past month, how long (in minutes) has it usually taken you to fall asleep at night?" (Buysse et al., 1989, p. 209).

SCORING: Detailed instructions for scoring appear in Buysse et al. (1989, pp. 211-213). The PSQI has 19 items for self-rating and five questions to be asked of a "bed partner or roommate." Only the self-rated items are considered when scoring. Scores for "the 19 items are combined to form seven component scores, each of which has a range of 0-3 points" (Buysse et al., 1989, p. 211). The global score, which is the sum of the seven component scores, has a range from 0 to 21. Higher PSQI scores indicate more sleep complaints. PSQI scores of 5 are suggested as cutoff points for "good sleepers."

SOURCE: The instrument is available from the author and also appears in the appendix to Buysse et al. (1989).

REFERENCES

Buysse, D. J., Reynolds, C. F., III, Monk, T. H., Berman, S. R., & Kupfer, D. J. (1989). The Pittsburgh Sleep Quality Index: A new instrument for psychiatric practice and research. *Psychiatry Research, 28,* 193-213.
Buysse, D. J., Reynolds, C. F., III, Monk, T. H., Hoch, C. C., Yeager, A. L., & Kupfer, D. J. (1991). Quantification of subjective sleep quality in healthy elderly men and women using the Pittsburgh Sleep Quality Index (PSQI). *Sleep, 14,* 331-338.

PLUTCHIK GERIATRIC RATING SCALE (GRS)

AUTHORS: R. Plutchik, Hope Conte, M. Leiberman, M. Bakur, J.
            Grossman, and N. Lehrman
ADDRESS: Hope R. Conte, PhD
            Director of Psychiatry
            Bronx Municipal Hospital Center, Residence, 2N8
            Pelham Parkway South and Eastchester Road
            Bronx, NY 10461

DESCRIPTION: The Plutchik Geriatric Rating Scale (GRS) is a 31-item scale designed to be completed by caregivers who are well acquainted with the subject. The GRS measures level of functioning in areas including activities of daily living, mobility, sensory abilities, sleep, confusion, communication, memory, social interaction, and disturbing behaviors (Plutchik et al., 1970).

PSYCHOMETRIC PROPERTIES: The GRS items, which are worded in brief, simple language, were judged by consensus to have content validity by a group of expert psychologists and psychiatrists. The subjects, when the instrument was initially tested, were 207 psychiatric patients in a state hospital. Their scores ranged from 0 to 51. The correlation for ratings assigned by two independent judges ($N = 86$) was 0.87 (Plutchik et al., 1970, p. 492). An item analysis was performed by comparing the scores of high- and low-functioning patients. Twenty-four items discriminated between the groups. Scores on 13 items about physical impairment and confusion discriminated between geriatric ($n = 50$) and nongeriatric ($n = 36$) patients; the mean GRS score for geriatric patients (23.92) was significantly different from the mean for nongeriatric patients (12.42; p. 497). In their study of the effects of special care units for Alzheimer's patients, Swanson, Maas, and Buckwalter (1994) found that scores on the Self-Care Abilities subscale of their Functional Abilities Checklist correlated (0.84) with GRS ratings made by residents' primary nurses (p. 34).

PROCEDURE: Raters who are familiar with the patient but require no special training circle one of three possible responses for each item.

SAMPLE ITEMS: "When bathing or dressing, the patient needs: No assistance = 0; Some assistance = 1; Maximum assistance = 2" and "The patient knows the name of: More than one member of the staff = 0; Only one member of the staff = 1; None of the staff = 2" (Plutchik et al., 1970, pp. 493-494).

SCORING: Each item is scored 0, 1, or 2. The sum of scores for the 31 items is considered a measure of overall level of functioning (Plutchik et al., 1970, p. 492). Higher scores indicate greater impairment.

SOURCE: Copies of the instrument appear in Plutchik et al. (1970) and Guy (1976).

REFERENCES

Guy, W. (1976). *Early Clinical Drug Evaluation Unit assessment manual for psychopharmacology* (Rev. ed., DHEW Pub. No. ADM 76-338). Washington, DC: Government Printing Office.

Plutchik, R., Conte, H., Leiberman, M., Bakur, M., Grossman, J., & Lehrman, N. (1970). Reliability and validity of a scale for assessing the functioning of geriatric patients. *Journal of the American Geriatrics Society, 18,* 232-237.

Swanson, E. A., Maas, M. L., & Buckwalter, K. C. (1994). Alzheimer's residents' cognitive and functional measures: Special and traditional care unit comparison. *Clinical Nursing Research, 3,* 27-41.

PREADMISSION ACUITY INQUIRY (PAI)

AUTHORS: Elizabeth A. Swanson and Orpha J. Glick
ADDRESS: Elizabeth A. Swanson, PhD, RN
             College of Nursing
             University of Iowa
             Iowa City, IA 52242

DESCRIPTION: The Preadmission Acuity Inquiry (PAI) was designed to assess level of dependence for the purpose of predicting care requirements for applicants to long-term care facilities. The authors conceptualized level of dependence as "acuity" (Swanson & Glick, 1995, p. 77). The PAI is divided into 21 major sections to assess "basic activities of daily living, the level of cognitive and sensory function, the past and current mental and physical illness and related treatments and the presence of maladaptive behavior" (p. 79). There are 97 items, which have been weighted by long-term care experts according to amount of care required. To facilitate use of the PAI by long-term care staff after a person is admitted, the items have the same sequence as the items in the Minimum Data Set (MDS) of the Resident Assessment Instrument (RAI; Morris et al., 1991).

PSYCHOMETRIC PROPERTIES: The Directors of Nursing (DONs) of eight long-term care facilities in Iowa classified their residents as "independent," "assist," or "dependent." Alphabetized lists were generated, and every fourth resident 65 or over "or their legally authorized other" was invited to participate in the validation study. There was a 24% refusal rate. Twelve nurse and social worker examiners, unaware of the resident's dependency category, interviewed 204 residents using the PAI; they also asked them to perform tasks for a Motor Performance Inventory (MPI) that had been designed for the study. Items for the MPI had been derived from the Direct Assessment of Functional Status (see entry in this book) and from Tinetti's (1986) Performance-Oriented Assessment of Mobility Problems. An estimate of interrater reliability was calculated for two independent assessments of every seventh participant. Means for agreement between raters (kappa) were 0.90 for the PAI and 0.91 for the MPI. Cronbach's alpha for the PAI was 0.81; for the MPI, it was 0.97. The instrument discriminated between the groups that had been classified by the DONs. The trend in mean PAI scores for the "independent" (27.3), "assist" (43.6) and "dependent" (72.5) groups ($F = 131.29$, $df = 2$, 196, $p < 0.0001$) supported concurrent validity. Correlations between self-report scores and performance scores for ADL components of the PAI and the MPI ranged between 0.62 and 0.82. With discriminant analysis, overall agreement between PAI scores and the DONs' classification was 60% (Swanson & Glick, 1995, p. 86), with the lowest agreement occurring in the "assist" category (17%). Residents had been placed in categories higher than they were actually able to demonstrate. The authors believe that the results of their "preliminary work demonstrate sufficient reliability and validity to merit further refinement and testing" (p. 87).

PROCEDURE: Data to complete the PAI are gathered by direct observation, as self-reports from the prospective resident, as reports of a "responsible other," or from health records. The PAI is designed to be used by nurses or social workers in an interview. Specific directions and suggested scripts are printed with items on the interview schedule.

SAMPLE ITEM:

> List Current Medication: [spaces are provided]. (This information can be obtained from the record or from observing the medication bottles. Review the current medication list and determine which of the scoring criteria below apply. Add each individual score to derive a total score.) Scoring criteria: 1 = 0-3 medications; 2 = 4-8 medications; 3 = administration with assessment (e.g., blood glucose, blood pressure, and pulse); 4 = injections/eye drops; 5 = psychotropics; 6 = topical skin treatments. (Swanson & Glick, 1990, p. 10) [There is a space provided for comments.]

SCORING: The PAI score is calculated by summing the "total scores" for the 21 sections of the instrument. The range for the PAI score is from 0 to

159+ (Swanson & Glick, 1995, p. 82). Scores higher than 159 would mean there had been observations of "maladaptive behaviors or required special treatment procedures" (p. 82).

SOURCE: The instrument is available from the authors, who hold a copyright.

REFERENCES

Morris, J. N., Hawes, C., Murphy, K., Nonemaker, S., Phillips, C. D., Fries, B. E., & Mor, V. (Eds.). (1991). *Resident Assessment Instrument training manual and resource guide.* Natwick, MA: Eliot.

Swanson, E. A., & Glick, O. J. (1990). *Preadmission Acuity Inquiry.* (Available from the authors at address listed above)

Swanson, E. A., & Glick, O. J. (1995). Reliability and validity of a new preadmission acuity tool for long-term care. *Journal of Nursing Measurement, 3,* 77-88.

Tinetti, M. E. (1986). Performance-oriented assessment of mobility problems in elderly patients. *Journal of the American Geriatrics Society, 34,* 119-126.

PULSES PROFILE (PULSES)

AUTHORS: Eugene Moskowitz and Cairbre McCann;
            adapted by Carl V. Granger

DESCRIPTION: Development of the PULSES Profile was first reported in 1957 by Moskowitz and McCann. PULSES scores reflected functional changes in aging and chronically disabled persons. PULSES was the acronym for six functional assessment categories: *P*hysical condition, *U*pper extremities, *L*ower extremities, *S*ensory, *E*xcretory, and mental and emotional *S*tatus. In each of these categories, there were descriptions of four functional levels. In 1979, Granger, Albrecht, and Hamilton reported a study in which a different PULSES format was used. They made five changes: (a) functional levels stressed independence (Levels 1 and 2) or need for assistance (Levels 3 and 4); (b) the "U" section referred to self-care activities as well as upper-extremity function; (c) "L" referred to mobility as well as to lower-extremity function; (d) the second "S" category was renamed "Support Factors," which included role performance, intellectual and emotional adaptability, family support, and financial ability; and (e) summation of subscores was suggested to yield a global score (p. 153). Moskowitz (1985), the originator of the scale, believed that when the six digits of PULSES were summed, information about the profile's six distinct categories was lost.

PSYCHOMETRIC PROPERTIES: The reliability and validity of the initial PULSES Profile were not reported by Moskowitz and McCann (1957). Granger et al. (1979) estimated test-retest reliability (0.87) and interscorer (0.95) reliability for their adapted version. They compared the PULSES and Barthel Index (see entry in this book) scores of 307 severely disabled rehabilitation patients and found that both instruments were "valid, reliable, and sensitive for describing functional abilities and change over a period of time" (p. 145).

PROCEDURE: The original profile was intended as an evaluation to be completed by a physician (Moskowitz & McCann, 1957, p. 343). According to Granger et al. (1979), staff can be trained to use the adapted version for both direct observation and medical record review (p. 647).

SAMPLE ITEM (Original Format):

S: Sensory components relating to speech, vision, and hearing.

1. No gross abnormalities considering the age of the individual.
2. Minor deviations insufficient to cause any appreciable functional impairment.
3. Moderate deviations sufficient to cause appreciable functional impairment.
4. Severe deviations causing complete loss of hearing, vision, or speech. (Moskowitz & McCann, 1957, p. 343)

SAMPLE ITEM (Adapted Version):

S: Sensory components relating to communication (speech and hearing) and vision.

1. Independent in communication and vision without impairment.
2. Independent in communication and vision with some impairment such as mild dysarthria, mild aphasia, or need for eyeglasses or hearing aid, or needing regular eye medication.
3. Dependent upon assistance, an interpreter, or supervision in communication or vision.
4. Dependent totally in communication or vision. (Granger et al., 1979, p. 153)

SCORING: In the original format, the PULSES score was the profile that included all six category scores recorded separately. Granger et al. (1979) suggested that PULSES scores be summed and that a global score of 12 was "a useful operational cutting point for distinguishing lesser from more marked disability, and 16 for indicating very severe disability" (p. 152).

SOURCE: The original PULSES Profile appears in Moskowitz and McCann (1957). A copy of the Granger et al. version is printed in the appendix to Granger et al. (1979). It is also reprinted in Matteson, McConnell, and Linton (1997).

REFERENCES

Granger, C. V., Albrecht, G. L., & Hamilton, B. B. (1979). Outcome of comprehensive medical rehabilitation: Measurement by PULSES Profile and the Barthel Index. *Archives of Physical Medicine and Rehabilitation, 60,* 145-154.

Matteson, M. A., McConnell, E. S., & Linton, A. D. (1997). *Gerontological nursing: Concepts and practice* (2nd ed.). Philadelphia: W. B. Saunders.

Moskowitz, E. (1985). PULSES Profile in retrospect. *Archives of Physical Medicine and Rehabilitation, 66,* 647.

Moskowitz, E., & McCann, C. B. (1957). Classification of disability in the chronically ill and ageing. *Journal of Chronic Disease, 5,* 342-346.

RAPID DISABILITY RATING SCALE-2 (RDRS2)

AUTHORS: Margaret W. Linn and Bernard S. Linn

DESCRIPTION: The Rapid Disability Rating Scale-2 (RDRS2) is a revised, 18-item version of the original Rapid Disability Rating Scale (Linn, 1967). Scale items address assistance with activities of daily living (ADLs) and instrumental activities of daily living, degree of disabilities, and degree of special problems such as confusion, uncooperativeness, and depression. Responses give a profile of how a subject is functioning at a particular point in time (Linn & Linn, 1982). The RDRS2 may be used to assess response to treatment, need for care, or level of disability.

PSYCHOMETRIC PROPERTIES: In validation studies, two nurses used the RDRS2 and rated 100 patients independently. Intraclass correlations for item ratings ranged from 0.62 (depression) to 0.98 (walking; sight). Correlations for test-retest reliabilities for item ratings of 50 patients at a 3-day interval ranged from 0.58 to 0.96. Validity of the scale was demonstrated with comparisons between RDRS2 scores and impairment ratings made by physicians and patient's self-reports (Linn & Linn, 1982, pp. 380-381).

PROCEDURE: The RDRS2 is designed to be completed by a family member, nurse, or nurse's aide who knows the subject. Respondents rate behaviors based on what the subject actually *does,* not on what he or she is capable of doing. The authors recommended one training session for the rater to improve reliability.

SAMPLE ITEM: Assistance with ADLs.

Grooming (shaving for men, hairdressing for women, nails, teeth)

| None | A little | A lot | Must be groomed |

(Linn & Linn, 1982, p. 380)

SCORING: Items are scored from *none* (1) to *severe* (4), with a range of total scores from 18 to 72. Scores of community dwelling elders with limited disability average 21 to 22. Hospitalized elderly persons score 32 on average, and those transferred to nursing homes have average scores of 36 (Linn & Linn, 1982, p. 380).

SOURCE: The instrument is reprinted in Linn (1988) and in Linn and Linn (1982).

REFERENCES

Linn, M. W. (1967). A rapid disability rating scale. *Journal of the American Geriatrics Society, 15,* 211-214.

Linn, M. W. (1988). Rapid Disability Rating Scale. *Psychopharmacology Bulletin, 24,* 799-800.

Linn, M. W., & Linn, B. S. (1982). The Rapid Disability Scale-2. *Journal of the American Geriatrics Society, 30,* 378-382.

RATING SCALE FOR AGGRESSIVE
BEHAVIOR IN THE ELDERLY (RAGE)

AUTHORS: Vikram Patel and R. A. Hope
ADDRESS: Dr. R. A. Hope
            Department of Psychiatry
            Warneford Hospital
            Oxford OX3 7JX, England

DESCRIPTION: The Rating Scale for Aggressive Behavior in the Elderly (RAGE) is a 21-item instrument designed for assessment of psychogeriatric patients by "ward-based nursing staff." The purpose of the RAGE was to facilitate research about the effects of treatment of aggressive behavior and to study the relationships between aggressive behavior and other factors (Patel & Hope, 1992, p. 211). The authors defined aggressive behavior as "an overt act, involving the delivery of noxious stimuli to (but not necessarily aimed at) another organism, object, self, which is clearly not accidental" (p. 212). Eighteen items relate to frequency of aggression, one to potential injury, and one to the use of restraint. The final item is a global assessment of aggression. The instrument has been translated into Spanish and Chinese.

PSYCHOMETRIC PROPERTIES: RAGE items were derived from clinical observations, interviews with caregivers, and the literature. They were piloted with 35 patients rated by two nurses. Nurses judged the scale as "simple to use . . . and relevant to the nursing problems in the management of dementia" (Patel & Hope, 1992, p. 213). Items with low item-to-total-score correlations were dropped from the scale. The 21 items selected were tested for a 3-day observation period with 90 inpatients on six psychogeriatric units in two hospitals. Nurses used their own observations, nursing notes, and change-of-shift reports as sources of data. In addition, in three of the six wards, another source of data was a ward checklist, a grid with patients' names on one axis and types of behavior on the other. All nursing staff on all shifts made notations on checklists. Ratings for aggression were far more reliable where the ward checklist had been used; Pearson r was 0.94 compared with 0.54. When ratings and checklists were compared, however, the improved reliability could not be attributed merely to nurses' having referred to the checklist. Test-retest reliability was estimated with independent observations for three time intervals: 6 hours, 7 days, and 14 days. Correlations for total scores at 6 hours was 0.91, with correlations for individual items ranging between 0.47 and 0.94. For the 7-day study, total score correlation was 0.84, with those for individual items ranging from 0.48 to 0.93. For the 14-day study, the correlation for total score was 0.88, and for items, the range was 0.5 to 1.00. The alpha coefficient for the scale was 0.89. Sensitivity was estimated by comparing independent serial observations of aggressive behavior with test-retest scores on the RAGE. Fourteen patients showed decreased aggression over time; their RAGE scores changed from 17.8 to 6.5. RAGE scores for seven patients with increased aggression changed from 6.7 to 16. Three factors identified for the RAGE were labeled Verbal Aggression, Physical Aggression, and Antisocial Behavior.

PROCEDURE: Preparation of raters is advised, and Patel and Hope (1992) provided specific suggestions. They recommended that the RAGE be used in conjunction with a ward checklist for rating aggressive behavior round the clock. "Instructions and Advice" for the rater are printed on the instrument. The major point stressed by the authors is that raters should be concerned *not* about the reasons, motives, or intent of aggression but *only* with the actual behaviors (p. 220).

SAMPLE ITEMS: "Has the patient in the last three days been demanding or argumentative?" and "Has the patient in the last three days attempted to hit others?" (Patel & Hope, 1992, p. 219).

SCORING: Responses to 18 of the items are rated 0 *(not once in the past three days)*, 1 *(at least once in the past three days)*, 2 *(at least once every day in the past three days)*, and 3 *(more than once every day in the past three days [always])*. Response choices for the other three items are described with the item (Patel & Hope, 1992, p. 219).

SOURCE: The instrument, with "Instructions and Advice," and guidelines for "Training for Raters," are printed in appendices to Patel and Hope (1992).

REFERENCE

Patel, V., & Hope, R. A. (1992). A rating scale for aggressive behavior in the elderly: The RAGE. *Psychological Medicine, 22,* 211-221.

RESILIENCE SCALE (RS)

AUTHORS: Gail M. Wagnild and Heather M. Young
ADDRESS: Gail M. Wagnild, RN, PhD
            Community Health Care Systems, SM-24
            School of Nursing
            University of Washington
            Seattle, WA 98195

DESCRIPTION: The authors of the Resilience Scale (RS) considered resilience "a positive personality characteristic that enhances individual adaptation" (Wagnild & Young, 1993, p. 167). The purpose of the scale is to identify the extent of an individual's resilience. The RS has 26 items designed to tap resilience as defined by five components: (a) equanimity, (b) perseverance, (c) self-reliance, (d) meaningfulness, and (e) existential aloneness. These components had been derived in a qualitative study of women who had been prescreened for positive psychosocial adaptation and characterized as resilient (Wagnild & Young, 1990).

PSYCHOMETRIC PROPERTIES: To construct the scale, the authors selected items from verbatim interview statements to reflect the instrument's five components. All items were positively worded. The scale was pilot-tested with samples of students, caregivers of spouses with Alzheimer's disease, first-time mothers returning to work, residents of public housing, and pregnant and postpartum women (Wagnild & Young, 1993, p. 168). Community-dwelling elders ($N = 810$) were surveyed with the RS and with other measures of adaptation. Concurrent validity was estimated with correlations between RS scores and scores on the Philadelphia Geriatric Center Morale Scale (0.28; see entry in this book), Life Satisfaction Index—A (0.30; Neugarten, Havighurst, & Tobin, 1961), Beck Depression Inventory (−0.37; see entry in this book), and self-rated health (−0.26; p. 174). Factor-analytic procedures led to a two-factor solution that explained 44% of the variance. Internal consistency for the RS has ranged between 0.76 and 0.91; item-to-total scale correlations ranged between 0.37 and 0.75 (p. 172). Test-retest reliability was estimated (range 0.67 to 0.84) from serial administrations of the RS to childbearing women (p. 173).

PROCEDURE: Respondents to the RS, a paper-and-pencil instrument, are asked to rate the extent of their agreement with 26 statements on a 7-point scale.

SAMPLE ITEMS: "My belief in myself gets me through hard times" and "I have enough energy to do what I have to do" (Wagnild & Young, 1993, p. 169).

SCORING: Each item is rated from 1 (*strongly disagree*) to 7 (*strongly agree*). Scores range from 26 to 182.

SOURCE: The scale is reproduced in Wagnild and Young (1993). The authors hold a copyright.

REFERENCES

Neugarten, B., Havighurst, R., & Tobin, S. (1961). The measure of life satisfaction. *Journal of Gerontology, 16,* 134-143.
Wagnild, G. M., & Young, H. M. (1990). Resilience among older women. *Image, 22,* 252-255.
Wagnild, G. M., & Young, H. M. (1993). Development and psychometric evaluation of the resilience scale. *Journal of Nursing Measurement, 1,* 165-178.

ROBERTS BALANCE SCALE (RBS)

AUTHOR: Beverly L. Roberts
ADDRESS: Beverly L. Roberts, PhD, RN
           Frances Payne Bolton School of Nursing
           Case Western Reserve University
           Cleveland, OH 44106-4904

DESCRIPTION: The Balance Scale developed by Roberts (RBS) has eight performance items. It was designed to meet the need for a portable measure of balance that could be administered to elders in clinical research settings. Based on the theory that base of support and visual cues are major factors related to balance, the scale tests four stances with the subject standing on the floor: "bipedal stance with eyes open and closed, monopedal stance with eyes open and closed" (Roberts & Mueller, 1987, p. 372). In addition, to "increase the sensitivity of the scale by stressing the mechanisms of balance control" (p. 372), subjects repeat the four stances while standing on a wooden beam 2 inches high and 3 inches wide.

PSYCHOMETRIC PROPERTIES: Earlier investigations (Roberts & Fitzpatrick, 1983) had supported content validity and stability of the scale. Construct validity and reliability of monopedal and bipedal stances as gauges of balance had been found in studies by other investigators. There was evidence also for the importance of visual cues as a factor in balance (Roberts & Mueller, 1987, p. 369). Roberts and Mueller (1987) studied balance in a sample of community-dwelling volunteer elders ($N = 61$) with mean age of 71.9 years. They were "healthy or had a well controlled chronic illness" (p. 370). There was "moderate" evidence supporting internal consistency (alpha = 0.82) of the scale (p. 372). Factor analysis revealed four factors different from those that had been expected theoretically. Although the authors stated that further testing was needed, they claimed that the results of their study supported construct validity.

PROCEDURE: Subjects are tested in their stocking feet. They place their hands on their hips for all stances. For the bipedal stance, feet are together and heels are off the floor. For the monopedal stance, the subject stands on one foot (chosen by the subject), "lifting the other foot off the ground by maximally flexing the knee" (Roberts & Mueller, 1987, p. 370). Two observers do the testing. One guards the subject to prevent falls, and the other observes the subject's feet and eyes to time the duration of the stance, using a stopwatch. Timing continues for 30 seconds or until the stance is broken or, in the closed-eyes condition, until the eyes are opened.

SCORING: The time the stance is maintained is the score for each stance.

SOURCE: The scale is available from the author.

REFERENCES

Roberts, B. L., & Fitzpatrick, G. G. (1983). Improving balance: Therapy of movement. *Journal of Gerontological Nursing, 9,* 151-156.

Roberts, B. L., & Mueller, M. G. (1987). The Balance Scale: Factor analysis and reliability. *Perceptual and Motor Skills, 65,* 367-374.

ROSENBERG SELF-ESTEEM SCALE (RSE)

AUTHOR: Morris Rosenberg

DESCRIPTION: The Rosenberg Self-Esteem Scale (RSE) is a 10-item instrument that can be used to estimate positive or negative feelings about the self (Blascovich & Tomaka, 1991, p. 123). It was originally conceived as a measure of the self-worth or self-acceptance in adolescents (Rosenberg, 1965). It has also been used widely with older adults (Linn, 1988) and is considered a standard against which other measures of self-esteem are evaluated (Blascovich & Tomaka, 1991, p. 123). Rosenberg (1979) linked the notions of self-esteem and self-concept theoretically. He defined self-concept as "the totality of the individual's thoughts and feelings with reference to himself as an object" (p. 7) and saw self-esteem as "the wish to think well of oneself" (p. 54).

PSYCHOMETRIC PROPERTIES: The RSE items have face validity and deal with a "general favorable or unfavorable global self-attitude" (Rosenberg, 1979, p. 292). The author's findings showed satisfactory coefficients for test-retest reliability, at 2 weeks, ranging from 0.85 to 0.88 (p. 292). Construct validity was supported with associations, in expected directions, between depression, anxiety, and sociometric ratings by peers. Convergent and discriminant validity for the measure were also validated in a study in which investigators used the multitrait-multimethod approach (Silber & Tippett, 1965).

PROCEDURE: Respondents are asked to strongly agree, agree, disagree, or strongly disagree with 10 statements. Five statements are positive and five are negative. The negative statements are scored in reverse.

SAMPLE ITEMS: "On the whole, I am satisfied with myself" and "I certainly feel useless at times" (Rosenberg, 1979, p. 291).

SCORING: Although it was designed as a Guttman scale, the SRE has also been scored in five-item and seven-item Likert scale formats.

SOURCE: The scale is reprinted in Rosenberg (1965, 1979).

REFERENCES

Blascovich, J., & Tomaka, J. (1991). Measures of self-esteem. In J. P. Robinson, P. R. Shaver, & L. S. Wrightsman (Eds.), *Measures of personality and social psychological attitudes* (pp. 115-160). San Diego: Academic Press.

Linn, M. W. (1988). A critical review of scales used to evaluate social and interpersonal adjustment in the community. *Psychopharmacology Bulletin, 24,* 615-621.

Rosenberg, M. (1965). *Society and the adolescent self-image.* Princeton, NJ: Princeton University Press.

Rosenberg, M. (1979). *Conceiving the self.* New York: Basic Books.

Silber, E., & Tippett, J. S. (1965). Self-esteem: Clinical assessment and measurement validation. *Psychological Reports, 16,* 1017-1071.

RYDEN AGGRESSION SCALES (RAS1 AND RAS2)

AUTHOR: Muriel B. Ryden

ADDRESS: Muriel B. Ryden, PhD, RN
            School of Nursing
            University of Minnesota
            308 Harvard Street Southeast, 6-101 Unit F
            Minneapolis, MN 55455-0342

DESCRIPTION: The Ryden Aggression Scales (RAS1 and RAS2) are designed to "assess the nature and frequency of occurrence of aggressive behavior" (Ryden, 1989, p. 1). They have been used with cognitively impaired adults living in both nursing homes and the community. The author defines aggression as "hostile action directed toward others, the environment, or the self" (p. 1). Aggression, according to the author's model, which was adapted from Lanza (1983), is manifested in three categories of behavior: physical, verbal, and sexual. The RAS1 is a 25-item Likert scale with three subscales: a 16-item Physically Aggressive Behavior subscale (PAB), a 4-item Verbally Aggressive Behavior subscale (VAB), and a 5-item Sexually Aggressive Behavior subscale (SAB). The RAS1 is used retrospectively by a respondent familiar with the subject. The RAS2, designed to be used prospectively, is a 26-item tally form, blocked for date and three 8-hour shifts, with the same subscales and behaviors, except that "pulling hair" was added to the PAB.

PSYCHOMETRIC PROPERTIES: The items for the scales were derived clinically and from the literature and were validated by nurse experts. Validity was supported by a comparison made between RAS scores and logs kept by caregivers. The RAS1 and RAS2 were used to document the aggressive behavior of cognitively impaired residents ($N = 124$) of four nursing homes. The instruments were completed independently by different observers. RAS1 scores correlated significantly (0.65) with RAS2 scores (Ryden, Bossenmaier, & McLachlan, 1991, p. 93). Internal consistency for the RAS1 was estimated at 0.88; for the three subscales, alpha coefficients were 0.74 (SAB), 0.90 (VAB), and 0.84 (PAB). Test-retest reliability for the RAS1, with data from a community sample ($N = 31$) at intervals of 8 to 12 weeks, was 0.86 (Ryden, 1989). Interrater agreement for the RAS2 was 0.88 (Ryden et al., 1991, p. 90).

PROCEDURE: The observer using the RAS1 rates a specific behavior listed on the scale as occurring *never, less than once a year, 1-11 times a year, 1-3 times a month, 1-6 times a week,* or *1 or more times daily.* There is additional space for the respondent to add and rate frequency of behaviors that are not included on the scale. With the RAS2, the observer records the number of times each listed behavior occurs on each shift on each day. The respondent may also be instructed to use an attached sheet to document a behavior in narrative form with the details of its context (Ryden et al., 1991, p. 90). The authors provided guidelines about what is and what is not aggressive behavior. There are specific instructions about sexually aggressive behaviors: "Behaviors are considered sexually aggressive only if they are against the expressed will and/or despite the resistance of the other person" (Ryden et al., 1991, p. 91).

SAMPLE ITEMS: PAB—"Scratching"; VAB—"Name calling"; SAB—"Hugging" (Ryden, 1989).

SCORING: Scores for frequency on the RAS1 range between 0 (*never*) and 5 (*1 or more times daily*). The RAS1 is scored by summing the rating for each of the 25 items. The RAS2 is scored by summing the number of aggressive behaviors observed within a given time period. A mean daily aggression score may be calculated with data from the RAS2.

SOURCE: The instruments and materials describing their development are available from the author.

REFERENCES

Lanza, M. (1983). Origins of aggression. *Journal of Psychosocial Nursing Mental Health Services, 12*(6), 11-16.

Ryden, M. B. (1989). *Description of the Ryden Aggression Scale.* (Available from the author at address listed above)

Ryden, M. B., Bossenmaier, M., & McLachlan, C. (1991). Aggressive behavior in cognitively impaired nursing home residents. *Research in Nursing and Health, 14,* 87-95.

SANDOZ CLINICAL ASSESSMENT-GERIATRIC (SCAG)

AUTHORS: Richard I. Shader, Jerold S. Harmatz, and Carl Salzman
ADDRESS: Richard I. Shader, MD
          Professor of Psychiatry and Professor of Pharmacology
              and Experimental Therapeutics
          Tufts University School of Medicine
          136 Harrison Avenue
          Boston, MA 02111

DESCRIPTION: The Sandoz Clinical Assessment-Geriatric (SCAG) was developed for use in psychopharmacological research with elderly persons (Shader, Harmatz, & Salzman, 1974). The SCAG consists of descriptions of 18 cognitive, affective, and behavioral symptoms and one global rating. It taps "five distinct domains of geriatric symptomatology: cognitive dysfunction, difficulties in interpersonal relationships, apathy, affect, and somatic dysfunction" (Hamot, Patin, & Singer, 1984, p. 147). The scale has been widely used to assess change in clinical trials. It has been shown to be a "consistently sensitive scale for differentiating active treatment from placebo" (Hamot et al., 1984, p. 142).

PSYCHOMETRIC PROPERTIES: The authors studied ratings made for a patient group ($n = 26$) and a control group ($n = 25$) of elders. The patient group included persons with affective disorders or severe dementia. The control group included persons described as healthy or as having mild dementia. The authors compared scores between and within groups. SCAG item scores for the patient group were significantly higher than those for the controls, except for the symptom of dizziness (Shader et al., 1974, p. 111). Depressed patients were differentiated from demented subjects on 7 of the

18 items of the scale (p. 112). Interrater reliability was tested with ratings made by four psychiatrists who observed the same clinical interviews of eight subjects. The average intraclass correlation coefficient was 0.75. The authors suggested that the extent of disagreement would have been "mitigated by training to criterion" (p. 112). Factor analyses by several investigators have shown highly consistent results (Overall & Rhoades, 1988).

PROCEDURE: The patient is interviewed by the clinician-rater. Using cues printed on the SCAG scale, the clinician rates the subject for the extent to which each symptom is present.

SAMPLE ITEM: "Fatigue: Sluggish, listless, tired, weary, worn out, bushed. Rate on patient's statements and observed response to normal daily activities outside interview situation" (Hamot et al., 1984, p. 144).

SCORING: Items are rated on a 7-point scale: *not present* (1), *very mild* (2), *mild* (3), *moderate* (4), *moderately severe* (5), *severe* (6), and *extremely severe* (7) (Hamot et al., 1984, p. 144). Scores for both individual items and factors are analyzed (p. 147).

SOURCE: A copy of the SCAG is reprinted in Hamot et al. (1984). There are also copies in Guy (1976) and in Shader, Harmatz, and Salzman (1988).

REFERENCES

Guy, W. (1976). *Early Clinical Drug Evaluation Unit assessment manual for psychophar-macology* (Rev. ed., DHEW Pub. No. ADM 76-338). Washington, DC: U.S. Department of Health, Education and Welfare.

Hamot, H. B., Patin, J. R., & Singer, J. M. (1984). Factor structure of the SCAG scale. *Psychopharmacology Bulletin, 20,* 142-150.

Overall, J. E., & Rhoades, H. M. (1988). Clinician-rated scales for multidimensional assessment of psychopathology in the elderly. *Psychopharmacology Bulletin, 24,* 587-594.

Shader, R. I., Harmatz, J. S., & Salzman, C. (1974). A new scale for assessment of geriatric populations: Sandoz Clinical Assessment-Geriatric (SCAG). *Journal of the American Geriatrics Society, 22,* 107-113.

Shader, R. I., Harmatz, J. S., & Salzman, C. (1988). Sandoz Clinical Assessment-Geriatric (SCAG). *Psychopharmacology Bulletin, 24,* 765-769.

SATISFACTION WITH LIFE SCALE (SWLS)

AUTHORS: Ed Diener, Robert A. Emmons, Randy J. Larsen,
             and Sharon Griffin
ADDRESS: Ed Diener, PhD, Professor
             Department of Psychology
             University of Illinois at Urbana-Champaign
             603 East Daniel Street
             Champaign, IL 61820

DESCRIPTION: The Satisfaction With Life Scale (SWLS) is a five-item measure of global life satisfaction intended for the general population. It focuses on the cognitive-judgmental aspects of subjective well-being and does not measure positive or negative affect. The tool has been used with diverse samples, including older adults. Items are written at 6th- to 10th-grade reading levels. Scores for most nonclinical groups, including elders, fall in the range of 23 to 28, "slightly satisfied" to "satisfied" (Pavot & Diener, 1993).

PSYCHOMETRIC PROPERTIES: Using factor analysis, the authors reduced their initial 48 items to 5. Internal consistency was tested with an undergraduate sample ($N = 176$) with an alpha coefficient of 0.87. Correlation for test-retest reliability ($N = 76$) with a 2-month interval was 0.82. The authors used principal-axis factor analysis; all five items loaded on a single factor and explained 66% of the variance (Diener, Emmons, Larsen, & Griffin, 1985, p. 72). Diener et al. (1985) showed that for a sample of elders ($N = 53$), SWLS scores were moderately correlated with interviewer ratings (0.44) and with scores on the Life Satisfaction Index (0.46; Adams, 1969). Among groups of prisoners, abused women, and psychiatric patients, SWLS scores were lower, as had been expected. SWLS scores were also reported to have changed following therapy and in conjunction with "good" and "bad" life events. The authors recommended supplementing the SWLS with other assessments (Pavot & Diener, 1993).

PROCEDURE: When the SWLS is administered, respondents are instructed to "be open and honest" as they indicate their agreement with the items on a scale from 1 to 7: 1 = *strongly disagree,* 2 = *disagree,* 3 = *slightly agree,* 4 = *neither agree nor disagree,* 5 = *slightly agree,* 6 = *agree,* and 7 = *strongly agree* (Diener et al., 1985).

ITEMS:

1. In most ways my life is close to my ideal.
2. The conditions of my life are excellent.
3. I am satisfied with my life.
4. So far I have gotten the important things I want in life.
5. If I could live my life over, I would change almost nothing. (Diener et al., 1985, p. 72)

SCORING: The range of scores is from 5 (low satisfaction) to 35 (high satisfaction). "A score of 20 represents the neutral point on the scale, the point at which the respondent is about equally satisfied and dissatisfied" (Pavot & Diener, 1993, p. 165). Scores for older adults gathered in several different studies (Total $N = 556$) have ranged between 19.7 and 27.9 (p. 166).

SOURCE: The instrument is in the public domain.

REFERENCES

Adams, D. L. (1969). Analysis of a life satisfaction index. *Journal of Gerontology, 24,* 470-474.
Diener, E., Emmons, R. A., Larsen, R. J., & Griffin, S. (1985). The Satisfaction With Life Scale. *Journal of Personality Assessment, 49,* 71-75.
Pavot, W., & Diener, E. (1993). Review of the Satisfaction With Life Scale. *Psychological Assessment, 5,* 164-171.

SELF-RATED HEALTH (SRH)

DESCRIPTION: Perceived health status, or self-ratings of health, have a "unique, predictive, and thus far inexplicable relationship with mortality" (Idler & Kasl, 1991, p. S64). They have been seen as "useful proxies" for clinically measured health status and as determinants of post-illness adjustment (Garrity, Somes, & Marx, 1978, p. 77). Self-rated health (SRH), as a single global measure, is easy and inexpensive to obtain. This measure has been proposed as a way to identify persons at increased risk for hospital admission or nursing home placement (Weinberger et al., 1986).

PSYCHOMETRIC PROPERTIES: Generally, moderate but significant correlations have been found between perceived health and findings on physical examination and physician ratings (Kaplan & Camacho, 1983, p. 293). Several studies with large U.S. and Canadian samples have shown that the way individuals view their health is related to subsequent health outcomes (Ferraro, 1980; Idler & Kasl, 1991; Kaplan & Camacho, 1983; Mossey & Shapiro, 1982). Ferraro (1980) analyzed cross-sectional data gathered in a population survey conducted by the U.S. Census Bureau ($N = 3,402$). In addition to SRH, the respondents, who were over 65 years old, provided "objective" health data by completing a disability scale and indicating their illnesses or physiological disorders on a checklist. Ferraro's results showed that both age and gender variables were important when considering SRH. "Old-old" (75 and older) persons with "excellent" SRH reported the same level of disability as the merely "old" (65 to 74) whose health had been rated "good" (p. 379). Males had a tendency to rate themselves as having poorer health, even though they reported fewer illnesses and disabilities (p. 380). Mossey and Shapiro (1982) studied SRH in a 6-year follow-up study ($N = 3,128$) conducted in Manitoba. With controls for "objective health status, age, gender, life satisfaction, income and urban/rural residence," they found that the risk of mortality was more than two times greater for persons whose SRH was "poor" than it was for those with an "excellent" SRH (p. 800). Kaplan and Camacho (1983) had similar results when they investigated the relationship between perceived health and mortality with another large sample ($N = 6,928$) followed up at 9 years. They estimated age-adjusted relative risk associated with "excellent" versus "poor" perceived health while controlling for other variables. Men and women with poor ratings had a 2.33 and a 5.10 greater mortality risk, respectively. The association was still apparent when the investigators controlled for effects of age, gender, initial physical status, health practices, social network participation, income, education, health relative to age peers, anomie, morale, depression, and happiness. These investigators speculated that individuals "may be able to access information" about the interactions between their "nervous, endocrine and immunological systems" and the "psychosocial influences on these interactions" (p. 302). The findings from these studies received further corroboration in another study. Idler and Kasl (1991) investigated the reasons for associations between expressions of subjective health status and survival. They did a 4-year follow-up of 2,812 persons over 65 who were participants in the Established Populations for the Epidemiological Study of the Elderly Project. Their findings were that "elderly persons whose perception of their health state is poor are as many as six times more likely to die than those who perceive their health as excellent" (p. S64). These investigators suggested that their findings should "engender new respect among health professionals for what people, especially the elderly people they treat, are saying about their health" (p. S65).

PROCEDURE: The question to generate a self-rating of health has been asked in slightly different ways by different investigators. Here are three examples.

1. "Compared to others your own age, how do you rate your health?" (Mossey & Shapiro, 1982, p. 800)
2. "All in all, would you say that your health is excellent, good, fair, or poor?" (Kaplan & Camacho, 1983, p. 294)
3. "Generally speaking, would you describe your present health as excellent (1), good (2), fair (3), or poor (4)?" (Ferraro, 1980, p. 378)

SCORING: Just as questions have varied, investigators have used different scoring systems for SRH.

REFERENCES

Ferraro, K. F. (1980). Self-ratings of health among the old and the old-old. *Journal of Health and Social Behavior, 21,* 377-383.

Garrity, T. F., Somes, G. W., & Marx, M. B. (1978). Factors influencing self-assessment of health. *Social Science and Medicine, 12,* 77-81.

Idler, E. L., & Kasl, S. (1991). Health perceptions and survival: Do global evaluations of health status really predict mortality? *Journal of Gerontology: Social Sciences, 46,* S55-S65.

Kaplan, G. A., & Camacho, T. (1983). Perceived health and mortality: A nine-year follow-up of the Human Population Laboratory cohort. *American Journal of Epidemiology, 117,* 292-304.

Mossey, J. M., & Shapiro, E. (1982). Self-rated health: A predictor of mortality among the elderly. *American Journal of Public Health, 72,* 800-808.

Weinberger, M., Darnell, J. C., Tierney, W. M., Martz, B. L., Hiner, S. L., Barker, J., & Neill, P. J. (1986). Self-rated health as a predictor of hospital admission and nursing home placement in elderly public housing tenants. *American Journal of Public Health, 76,* 457-459.

SERENITY SCALE (SERENITY)

AUTHOR: Kay T. Roberts
ADDRESS: Kay T. Roberts, EdD, RN
            Professor of Nursing
            University of Louisville
            3696 Webb Road
            Simpsonville, KY 40067

DESCRIPTION: The Serenity Scale is a 40-item tool designed to "evaluate serenity status" (Roberts & Aspy, 1993, p. 145). Items for the scale were selected to reflect the 10 "critical attributes" derived in a concept analysis of serenity (Roberts & Fitzgerald, 1991). The "critical attributes" central to the author's definition of the concept include

(1) The ability to be in touch with an inner haven of peace and security; (2) The ability to detach from excessive desires and emotions; (3) The ability to accept situations that cannot be changed; (4) The habit of actively pursuing all reasonable avenues for solving problems; (5) The ability to let go of the past, not worry about the future, and to live in the present; (6) Forgiveness of self and others; (7) A sense of connectedness and belonging; (8) Giving of one's self unconditionally; (9) A trust in a power greater than one's self; (10) A sense of perspective of the importance of one's self and life events. (Roberts & Aspy, 1993, pp. 147-148)

PSYCHOMETRIC PROPERTIES: Each item in an initial pool was rated by experts for its ability to yield information about serenity. The instrument, in its initial 65-item version, was tested first with 44 graduate students (mean age = 35), and 95 older adults (mean age = 75) who resided at two "congregate living" sites. Alpha coefficients for scores from these samples ranged between 0.92 and 0.95. The scale was revised and tested further with a volunteer sample ($N = 542$) structured to be diverse and representative for age, race, income, and health status. Data gathered from this sample were used to shorten the instrument. Internal consistency for the 40-item tool was 0.92. Item-to-total scale correlations ranged from 0.29 to 0.67. Factor analysis resulted in nine factors that were "logically congruent with the critical attributes of serenity" (Roberts & Aspy, 1993, p. 158) and "explained 58.2%

of the variance" (p. 154). Individuals with low literacy skills and education levels had some difficulties completing the tool (p. 154).

PROCEDURE: Respondents are instructed to complete the item without thinking about it too long. They are asked to evaluate the frequency of their experience of the "thoughts, feelings and actions" (Roberts & Aspy, 1993, p. 161) described in the item statement. The instrument takes from 12 to 30 minutes to complete.

SAMPLE ITEMS: "I experience peace of mind," "I find ways to share my talents with others," and "I feel resentful" (Roberts & Aspy, 1993, pp. 161-164).

SCORING: For each item, the respondent circles a number between 1 (*never*) and 5 (*always*). Assuming that all items are completed, scores range from 40 to 200. Twelve items are scored in reverse.

SOURCE: The scale is printed in the appendix to Roberts and Aspy (1993). Its copyright is held by the *Journal of Nursing Measurement.*

REFERENCES

Roberts, K. T., & Aspy, C. B. (1993). Development of the Serenity Scale. *Journal of Nursing Measurement, 1,* 145-164.
Roberts, K. T., & Fitzgerald, L. (1991). Serenity: Caring with perspective. *Scholarly Inquiry for Nursing Practice: An International Journal, 5,* 127-146.

SESSING SCALE (SS)

AUTHORS: Bruce A. Ferrell, Barbara M. Artinian, and Daphne Sessing
ADDRESS: Bruce A. Ferrell, MD
            Geriatric Research Education and Clinical Center
            Sepulveda VA Medical Center (11E)
            16111 Plummer Street
            Sepulveda, CA 91343

DESCRIPTION: The Sessing Scale was designed to measure progress in wound healing over time. It is a 7-point categorical scale with descriptions of skin, granulation tissue, infection, drainage, odor, necrosis, and eschar (Ferrell, Artinian, & Sessing, 1995).

PSYCHOMETRIC PROPERTIES: The language for the Sessing Scale was derived from descriptive statements made by a nurse who is an expert in wound care. Early versions of the scale were tested in a pilot study. Items were clarified "until the score assigned to a patient matched the expert's clinical sense of how the healing process was progressing" (Ferrell et al., 1995, p. 38). Five expert judges who were clinical specialists in wound care evaluated the scale for its "conceptual framework, content and hierarchy" (p. 38). Content validity was demonstrated by their consensus (100%). In three long-term care settings, 84 residents with pressure ulcers of the trunk or trochanter were evaluated twice weekly by nurses using the Shea Scale (Shea, 1975) and the Sessing Scale "until their wounds healed or they died or were transferred" (pp. 38-39). Average diameters of the ulcers were computed (square root of surface area), and concurrent validity for the Sessing Scale was demonstrated by relationships between average diameters and the Sessing Scale score (0.65), and between Sessing Scale scores and Shea Scale scores (0.90). Test-retest reliability (weighted kappa = 0.90) and interrater reliability (weighted kappa = 0.80) were tested by expert nurses with small subgroups of patients ($ns = 10$).

PROCEDURE: The observer assigns "the numerical value associated with the description that most closely matches the observed pressure ulcer" (Ferrell et al., 1995, p. 39).

SAMPLE ITEM: "Wound bed filling with pink granulating tissue" (Ferrell et al., 1995, p. 39).

SCORING: Scores assigned range from 0 to 6.

SOURCE: The scale is available from the authors. It is reprinted in Ferrell et al. (1995).

REFERENCES

Ferrell, B. A., Artinian, B. M., & Sessing, D. (1995). The Sessing Scale for assessment of pressure ulcer healing. *Journal of the American Geriatrics Society, 43,* 37-40.

Shea, D. J. (1975). Pressure sores classification and management. *Clinical Orthopedics, 112,* 89-100.

SICKNESS IMPACT PROFILE (SIP)

AUTHORS: Marilyn Bergner and Ruth A. Bobbitt, with Shirley
            Kressel, William E. Pollard, Betty S. Gilson, and Joanne
            R. Morris
ADDRESS: Department of Health Services, SC-37
            University of Washington
            Seattle, WA 98195

DESCRIPTION: The Sickness Impact Profile (SIP) is a 136-item behaviorally based measure designed to determine the respondent's perceived health status. It is a measure of sickness-related functional impairment that can be divided into physical and psychosocial dimensions. There are 12 categories of data: (a) body care and movement, (b) mobility, (c) ambulation, (d) emotional behavior, (e) social interaction, (f) alertness behavior, (g) communication, (h) sleep and rest, (i) home management, (j) work, (k) recreation and pastimes, and (l) eating. The SIP was developed to be "sensitive enough to detect changes or differences in health status that occur over time or between groups" (Bergner, Bobbitt, Carter, & Gibson, 1981, p. 787). The intention of the authors was "to provide a measure of the effects or outcomes of health care that can be used for evaluation, program planning and policy formulation" (Bergner et al., 1981, p. 787). The SIP has been used extensively with diverse samples. Rothman, Hedrick, and Inui (1989) found that it could be used with a nursing home sample as a comprehensive assessment of physical function. Gerety et al. (1994) reduced the number of items in the SIP to construct a Sickness Impact Profile for Nursing Homes.

PSYCHOMETRIC PROPERTIES: The instrument was developed, tested, revised, and refined in a comprehensive painstaking process (Bergner et al., 1976, 1981). Test-retest reliability (0.92) and internal consistency (0.94) for field trials with large samples demonstrated reliability. Validity was supported with correlations between SIP scores and self-assessments, clinician ratings, and scores on the National Health Interview Survey of Activity Limitation, Work Loss, and Bed Days. Clinical validity was substantiated with support for hypotheses about specific clinical measures and SIP scores (Bergner et al.,

1981, p. 798). Persons in particular diagnostic groups (e.g., hip replacement) showed "a consistent pattern of dysfunction across all patients and all administrations of the SIP" (p. 800). Gerety et al. (1994) noted that an important characteristic of the SIP is its ability to detect change in function in individuals over time.

PROCEDURE: The SIP may be self-administered or administered in an interview (Bergner et al., 1981, p. 788). Respondents are asked to check only those statements that apply to them on a given day.

SAMPLE ITEMS: "I walk shorter distances or stop to rest often," "I isolate myself as much as I can from the rest of my family," and "I am eating special or different food" (Bergner et al., 1981, p. 789).

SCORING: Separate scores may be calculated for the overall SIP and for the physical and psychosocial dimensions. SIP items have predetermined weights signifying a standardized evaluation for each dysfunction statement. The higher the score, the greater the disability. The overall SIP percent score is "obtained by summing the scale values of all items endorsed in the entire SIP, dividing that sum by the sum of the values of all the items in the SIP and multiplying the obtained quotient by 100" (Bergner et al., 1981, p. 790). Scores for the 12 categories may be computed in a similar way.

SOURCE: The instrument and supporting materials are available from the Department of Health Services, University of Washington, at the above address.

REFERENCES

Bergner, M., Bobbitt, R. A., Carter, W. B., & Gibson, B. S. (1981). The Sickness Impact Profile: Development and final revision of a health status measure. *Medical Care, 191*, 787-805.
Bergner, M., Bobbitt, R. A., Kressel, S., Pollard, W. E., Gilson, B. S., & Morris, J. R. (1976). The Sickness Impact Profile: Conceptual formulation and methodology for the development of a health status measure. *International Journal of Health Services, 6*, 393-415.
Gerety, M., Cornell, J. E., Mulrow, C. D., Tuley, M., Hazuda, H. P., Lichtenstein, M., Aguilar, C., Kadri, A., & Rosenberg, J. (1994). The Sickness Impact Profile for Nursing Homes (SIP-NH). *Journal of Gerontology, Medical Sciences, 49*, M2-M8.
Rothman, M. L., Hedrick, S., & Inui, T. (1989). The Sickness Impact Profile as a measure of the health status of noncognitively impaired nursing home residents. *Medical Care, 27*(3, Suppl.), 157-167.

SICKNESS IMPACT PROFILE FOR NURSING HOMES (SIP-NH)

AUTHORS: Meghan B. Gerety, John E. Cornell, Cynthia D. Mulrow,
            Michael Tuley, Helen P. Hazuda, Michael Lichtenstein,
            Christine Aguilar, Abdulhay A. Kadri, and Jeff Rosenberg
ADDRESS: Meghan B. Gerety, MD
            Audie L. Murphy Memorial Veterans Hospital
            7400 Merton Minter Boulevard, 11C6
            San Antonio, TX 78284

DESCRIPTION: The Sickness Impact Profile for Nursing Homes (SIP-NH) is a 66-item measure of self-perceived quality of life for nursing home residents. The tool is an adaptation of the Sickness Impact Profile (SIP; see entry in this book). The SIP-NH was designed to reduce respondent burden and to eliminate items that were not applicable to the nursing home population. There are physical disability and psychosocial subscales. The 10 categories of inquiry are (a) sleep and rest, (b) emotional behavior, (c) body care and movement, (d) mobility, (e) social interaction, (f) ambulation, (g) alertness behavior, (h) communication, (i) recreation/pastimes, and (j) eating. Two categories in the original SIP—work and home management—were eliminated.

PSYCHOMETRIC PROPERTIES: Using data from a sample of ethnically diverse, cognitively intact nursing home residents ($N = 231$), the authors used several methods to delete SIP items. Their goal was to retain the statistical integrity of the SIP and at the same time to improve the clinical relevance of the instrument. A team of experts made decisions to remove items if they "were likely to represent the inherent restrictions of the nursing home environment rather than the subject's illness-related disability" (Gerety et al., 1994, p. M3). Items with low item-to-total scale correlations and with relatively small contributions to the alpha coefficients were also deleted. The resulting 66-item instrument had psychometric properties similar to those of the original SIP. Correlations between SIP-NH scores and SIP scores and scores on validating instruments supported the validity of the shortened scale (p. M6). Gerety stated that it was not yet clear whether the SIP-NH was capable of measuring change (p. M8).

PROCEDURE: The instrument is designed to be completed in an interview. Each section of items is introduced with a prescribed general statement. Respondents are instructed, "Please respond TRUE if the statement describes you today. Respond NOT TRUE if the statement does not describe you today." If the answer is TRUE, the respondent is also asked, "Is that related to your health or because you are in a nursing home?" (Gerety, 1995).

SAMPLE ITEM: "I get around in a wheelchair. Is that true or not true? If true, is that related to your health or because you are in a nursing home?" (Gerety, 1995).

SCORING: Scoring the SIP-NH is a complex process. The interviewer records two scores for each item. The authors have retained the standardized weighting of items originally established for the SIP. Computations of total scores, scores for the subscales, and scores for each of the 10 categories are handled with a computer program. An SAS scoring program, SIPSCORE, is available with the instrument from the authors.

SOURCE: The SIP-NH is available from the authors.

REFERENCES

Gerety, M. (1995). *Sickness Impact Profile—Nursing Home Version.* (Available from the author at address listed above)

Gerety, M., Cornell, J. E., Mulrow, C. D., Tuley, M., Hazuda, H. P., Lichtenstein, M., Aguilar, C., Kadri, A., & Rosenberg, J. (1994). The Sickness Impact Profile for Nursing Homes (SIP-NH). *Journal of Gerontology, Medical Sciences, 49,* M2-M8.

SITUATIONAL CONTROL OF DAILY ACTIVITIES SCALE (SCDA)

AUTHOR: Betty L. Chang
ADDRESS: Betty L. Chang
            School of Nursing
            University of California, Los Angeles
            10833 Le Conte Avenue
            Los Angeles, CA 90024-1702

DESCRIPTION: The Situational Control of Daily Activities Scale (SCDA) was developed for use with elderly persons residing in institutions. It measures "patient perception of situational control" (Chang, 1978, p. 183). The original version of the instrument was open-ended and designed to be completed in an interview. Items in the early tool are phrased "Who determines that?" The latest version is a Likert scale with 34 items in nine categories: (a) ambulating, (b) dressing, (c) eating, (d) grooming, (e) toileting, (f) treatments, (g) group participation, (h) one-to-one interaction, and (i) solitary activities (Chang, 1995). Items in the new tool require the respondent to rate degree of self-determination for each item from 1 (*all the time by myself*) to 5 (*all the time by others*).

PSYCHOMETRIC PROPERTIES: Information about reliability and validity are published for the early version. The tool was administered during interviews with residents (*N* = 79) of eight nursing homes. Responses to items were rated either self-determined or other-determined. The correlation for test-retest reliability at a 3-month interval (*N* = 20) was 0.96. Interrater reliability (1.0) was determined by having every fifth interview coded independently by two observers (Chang, 1978, p. 184). Factor analysis showed two dimensions, with "Control of Physical Care" being distinguished from "Control of Socializing and Privacy." Grooming loaded on both factors. Ryden (1985), who used the tool in a nursing home study about environmental support for autonomy, modified the SCDA to create a "staff version" of the instrument. She inquired of staff about the reality of their situations and also about their preference for situational control.

PROCEDURE: The instrument may be administered as a paper-and-pencil test or completed in an interview.

SAMPLE ITEMS: "To what extent do I determine when I eat?" and "To what extent do I decide whether to participate in group activities?" (Chang, 1995).

SCORING: Chang reported means for her sample for the eight categories. Overall scores were considered "self-determined" if responses to five or more categories were self-determined or when there was a four-to-four tie (Chang, 1978, p. 184).

SOURCE: The new instrument (Chang, 1995) is available from the author, who holds its copyright. The early version appears as an appendix to Chang (1978).

REFERENCES

Chang, B. L. (1978). Perceived situational control of daily activities: A new tool. *Research in Nursing and Health, 1,* 181-188.

Chang, B. L. (1995). *The Situational Control of Daily Activities Scale.* (Available from the author at address listed above)

Ryden, M. B. (1985). Environmental support for autonomy in the institutionalized elderly. *Research in Nursing and Health, 8,* 363-371.

SIX-MINUTE WALKING TEST (SMWT)

AUTHORS: Gordon H. Guyatt, Michael J. Sullivan,
            Penelope J. Thompson, Ernest L. Fallen,
            Stewart O. Pugsley, D. Wayne Taylor, and
            Leslie B. Berman

ADDRESS: Dr. Gordon H. Guyatt
            Department of Clinical Epidemiology and Biostatistics
            McMaster University
            1200 Main Street W, Room 2C12
            Hamilton, Ontario L8N 3Z5, Canada

DESCRIPTION: The 6-minute walk, a performance test of functional exercise capacity, measures the distance walked in 6 minutes, after two trials. It is a simple, inexpensive, and safe test in which the subject controls the rate of exercise. Walking tests, which have been found acceptable to frail elderly persons, correspond to everyday functional activity. The 6-minute walk approximates "the usual day-to-day activity of moderately to severely limited patients" (Guyatt et al., 1985, p. 920). It can be used to monitor clinical progress and as an outcome measure to test the effectiveness of interventions.

PSYCHOMETRIC PROPERTIES: Walking test scores have generally correlated well with other functional measures (Morgan, Peck, Buchanan, & Hardy, 1983). Guyatt et al. (1985) walked ambulatory care patients, 18 with chronic heart failure and 25 with chronic lung disease, to test the effectiveness of a 6-minute walking test. Subjects walked six times at 2-week intervals. Scores for the 6-minute walk were correlated (low to moderate) with scores for functional tests (Specific Activities Scale and Functional Classification of the New York Heart Association; Goldman, Hashimoto, Cook, & Loscalzo, 1981) and results of maximal exercise testing using ergometer bicycles. Both patient groups showed improvement in scores up to the third walk, and scores on the test were stable thereafter. Encouragement of walkers significantly improved performance in both the cardiac and chronic lung disease groups.

PROCEDURE: In an area where the distance has been premeasured (Guyatt et al., 1985, used a 33-meter corridor), subjects are given instructions something like "This hall is _____ meters (or feet) long. I want you to walk back and forth as many times as you can before I say: stop. Start walking now." The stopwatch is kept inconspicuous. Assuming that protocol includes standardized encouragement, at 30-second intervals, say something like "Keep up the good work," "You're doing well," or "That's very good." At the end of 6 minutes, the tester calls out, "Stop," and the distance is recorded (Guyatt et al., 1985, p. 920).

SCORING: The test area is premeasured. The subject completes two trials. The investigator times the walk with a stopwatch and notes distance traveled by the subject in 6 minutes.

SOURCE: The procedure is specified in the article describing the test (Guyatt et al., 1985).

REFERENCES

Goldman, L., Hashimoto, B., Cook, E. F., & Loscalzo, A. (1981). Comparative reproducibility and validity of systems for assessing cardiovascular functional class: Advantages of a new specific activity scale. *Circulation, 64,* 1227-1234.

Guyatt, G. H., Sullivan, M. J., Thompson, P. J., Fallen, E. L., Pugsley, S. O., Taylor, D. W., & Berman, L. B. (1985). The 6-minute walk: A new measure of exercise capacity in patients with chronic heart failure. *Canadian Medical Association Journal, 132,* 919-923.

Morgan, A. D., Peck, D. F., Buchanan, D. R., & Hardy, G. J. R. (1983). Effects of attitudes and beliefs on exercise tolerance in chronic bronchitis. *British Medical Journal, 286,* 171-173.

SOCIAL DISABILITY QUESTIONNAIRE (SDQ)

AUTHORS: Laurence G. Branch and Alan M. Jette
ADDRESS: Laurence G. Branch, PhD
            Duke University Center on Aging
            Box 3003
            Durham, NC 27710

DESCRIPTION: The Social Disability Questionnaire (SDQ) was used in the Framingham Disability Study, which was part of the epidemiological study about heart disease conducted in Framingham, Massachusetts. The authors conducted the Disability Study to "investigate the nature and magnitude of disability among noninstitutionalized aging adults" (Branch & Jette, 1981, p. 1202). They defined social disability as "limitation in or inability to perform social roles or obligations" (p. 1202). The SDQ is composed of five indexes related to needs for independent living: (a) housekeeping, (b) transportation, (c) social interaction, (d) food preparation, and (e) grocery shopping. The authors were concerned with identifying unmet needs. They made a distinction between "need for assistance" and "unmet need for assistance." The person who has a need for assistance may also have the support necessary to meet the need. It is the person who does not have the support to meet the need "whose quality of life or independence is in immediate jeopardy" (p. 1203). The unmet needs for assistance are defined operationally by responses to the SDQ.

PSYCHOMETRIC PROPERTIES: The social disability measures had been used originally in an earlier survey conducted by Branch (1977) in Massachusetts. In the Framingham study, 2,654 surviving members of a noninstitutionalized cohort responded to the SDQ. Branch and Jette (1981) showed that the percentage of people needing or at risk of needing assistance to perform their social roles was a function of age (pp. 1206-1207).

PROCEDURE: The instrument can be used for in-person interviews or on the telephone.

SAMPLE ITEM: IV. Food Preparation Need.

> Who usually does the cooking? 1 = *Self,* 2 = *Household member,* 3 = *Someone outside the household.*
>
> If you had to, could you do all the cooking yourself? 1 = *Yes,* 2 = *No, for reason other than old age or illness,* 3 = *No, because of illness.*
>
> At the present time, does getting the food prepared usually give you: 1 = *No difficulty,* 2 = *A little difficulty,* 3 = *A lot of difficulty.*
>
> Not counting the times you might snack, how many regular meals do you usually have? 1 = *One,* 2 = *Two,* 3 = *Three or more.*
>
> Are there times when you do not eat enough of the right kind of food? 1 = *No,* 2 = *Once in a while,* 3 = *Sometimes,* 4 = *Often.* (Branch & Jette, 1981, p. 1209)

The food preparation need index combines descriptive information on who prepares meals, could the respondent prepare meals if necessary, frequency of eating the right kind of food and the number of regular meals each day, with evaluative information on the level of difficulty in getting food prepared. Unmet food preparation need is ascribed to an individual reporting only one regular meal a day, cannot prepare one's own food, sometimes or often does not eat the right kind of food, and reports a lot of difficulty with food preparation. (pp. 1209-1210)

SCORING: Respondents to the SDQ can be grouped into one of four categories using specific scoring logic for each index: "1 = *need met, no apparent problem;* 2 = *need met, potential problem;* 3 = *uncertain need met, potential problem;* 4 = *need unmet, current problem*" (Branch & Jette, 1981, p. 1203).

SOURCE: Branch and Jette (1981) provided copies of their items and the logic for computing the scoring algorithm. Branch (1977, 1980) published the exact operational definitions used in the needs assessment.

REFERENCES

Branch, L. G. (1977). *Understanding the health and social service needs of people over age 65.* Cambridge: Center for Survey Research of the University of Massachusetts and the Joint Center for Urban Studies of Massachusetts Institute of Technology and Harvard University.

Branch, L. G. (1980). *Vulnerable elders* (Gerontological Monograph No. 6). (Available from the Gerontological Society of America, 1275 K Street, NW, Suite 350, Washington, DC 20005-4006)

Branch, L. G., & Jette, A. M. (1981). The Framingham Disability Study: I. Social disability among the aging. *American Journal of Public Health, 71,* 1202-1210.

SPIRITUAL WELL-BEING SCALE (SWBS)

AUTHORS: Raymond F. Paloutzian and Craig W. Ellison
ADDRESS: Raymond F. Paloutzian
            Professor of Psychology
            Westmont College
            955 La Paz Road
            Santa Barbara, CA 93108-1099

DESCRIPTION: The Spiritual Well-Being Scale (SWBS) is a 20-item measure of the perceived spiritual quality of life developed to indicate general subjective well-being. There are two subscales: the Religious Well-Being Scale (RWBS) and the Existential Well-Being Scale (EWBS). The authors referred to the scale as "nonsectarian." Half the items include the word *God* (RWBS), and the other half do not (EWBS). The instrument was normed with volunteer samples in the Pacific Northwest and has been used by more than 300 investigators and clinicians with church, student, seminary, patient, and sociopathic convict samples (Paloutzian & Ellison, 1991). The authors cautioned users that scores from samples tested have not been distributed normally (Bufford, Paloutzian, & Ellison, 1991). Scores for religious samples were very high. The authors stated that the scale "appears to be most useful in clinical settings to detect the presence of a significantly impaired level of well-being" (p. 66).

PSYCHOMETRIC PROPERTIES: Results from the investigation of test-retest reliability of SWBS and its subscales at 1- to 10-week intervals ranged between 0.73 and 0.99 (Bufford et al., 1991). Internal consistency with alpha coefficients ranging from 0.82 to 0.94 (RWBS), 0.78 to 0.86 (EWBS), and 0.89 to 0.94 (SWBS) has also been demonstrated. Scores on the SWBS conform to expected values for known groups. Validity is also supported by positive correlations with scores for "positive self concept, finding meaning and purpose in life, high assertiveness and low aggressiveness, good physical health, and good emotional adjustment" (p. 57).

PROCEDURE: The instrument may be self-administered as a paper-and-pencil test or used orally. Completion takes 10 to 15 minutes.

SAMPLE ITEMS: "I believe that God loves me and cares about me" and "I feel very fulfilled and satisfied with life" (Paloutzian & Ellison, 1982, p. 233).

SCORING: Specific directions to score the items and norms are provided in the manual for the scale.

SOURCE: The instrument is copyrighted and available with a manual from the authors, with the understanding that users inform them about findings.

REFERENCES

Bufford, R. K., Paloutzian, R. F., & Ellison, C. W. (1991). Norms for the Spiritual Well-Being Scale. *Journal of Psychology and Theology, 19,* 56-70.

Paloutzian, R. F., & Ellison, C. W. (1982). Loneliness, spiritual well-being and quality of life. In L. A. Peplau & D. Perlman (Eds.), *Loneliness: A sourcebook of current theory, research, and therapy* (pp. 224-237). New York: Wiley-Interscience.

Paloutzian, R. F., & Ellison, C. W. (1991). *Manual for the Spiritual Well-Being Scale (Version 1.0).* (Available from the authors at address listed above)

STOKES/GORDON STRESS SCALE (SGSS)

AUTHORS: Shirlee A. Stokes and Susan E. Gordon
ADDRESS: Stokes/Gordon Stress Study
             Pace University
             Lienhard School of Nursing
             861 Bedford Road
             Pleasantville, NY 10570

DESCRIPTION: The Stokes/Gordon Stress Scale (SGSS) is a 104-item scale developed specifically for use with adults 65 and older. Members of several convenience samples who participated in instrument development (Stokes & Gordon, 1988) were residents of Florida or suburbs of New York City and were "healthy," defined as "residing in their own homes, able to care for themselves, and able to leave their homes as desired" (p. 17). Therefore, the scale is appropriate for use only with selected long-term clients and family members. Items on the scale reflect both major life events and everyday hassles.

PSYCHOMETRIC PROPERTIES: Items were "drawn from the literature, suggested by individuals 65 and over, and reviewed by two experts in gerontologic nursing" (Stokes & Gordon, 1988, p. 17). Items were ranked and weighted by a sample of older persons ($n = 43$) using a Q-sort procedure. Concurrent validity was established with significant correlations between SGSS scores ($n = 11$) and scores on two other life event scales ($r = 0.81$ and $r = 0.65$). Some support for the predictive ability of the scale was demonstrated with a correlation (0.36, $p = .014$) between SGSS scores ($n = 46$) and number of entries in health diaries indicating onset of illness, defined as "a visit to a health professional for reasons other than health maintenance"

(p. 18). Test-retest reliability was measured with three small samples at a 2-week interval, with correlations of 0.98, 0.91, and 0.90. Internal consistency ($n = 63$) with an alpha coefficient of 0.86 was also reported.

PROCEDURE: The scale is designed to be administered in person or by mail. Directions for subjects are written on the top of the scale itself. The scale takes 15 to 30 minutes to complete.

SAMPLE ITEMS: "Change in ability to do own personal care" and "Fear of being a victim of a street crime" (Stokes & Gordon, 1988, p. 18).

SCORING: An investigator or clinician needs information about item weights to calculate the stress score. The score is the sum of the weights for individual items checked by the respondent.

SOURCE: The scale and the user's manual, which includes a list of ranked item weights and a scoring sheet designed for convenient use, may be obtained from the author.

REFERENCE

Stokes, S. A., & Gordon, S. E. (1988). Development of an instrument to measure stress in the older adult. *Nursing Research, 37,* 16-19.

SYMPTOM DISTRESS SCALE (SDS)

AUTHORS: Ruth McCorkle and Katherine Young
ADDRESS: Ruth McCorkle, PhD, RN, Director
             Center for Advancing Care in Serious Illness
             School of Nursing, University of Pennsylvania
             420 Guardian Drive
             Philadelphia, PA 19104

DESCRIPTION: The Symptom Distress Scale (SDS) is an instrument to measure the degree of patient-perceived distress due to "nausea (presence and intensity), appetite, insomnia, pain (presence and intensity), fatigue, bowel patterns, concentration, dyspnea, appearance, outlook, and cough" (McCorkle et al., 1994, p. 245). Originally, the SDS was a 10-item tool designed "to identify concerns of patients receiving active cancer treatments" (McCorkle, 1987, p. 254). It has since been used with other chronically ill populations in a variety of settings. The original scale (McCorkle & Young, 1978) has been modified in both content and format.

PSYCHOMETRIC PROPERTIES: Alpha coefficients to measure internal consistency of the scale have ranged from 0.70 to 0.89 (McCorkle, 1987, p. 254; McCorkle et al., 1994, p. 245). The author reported that SDS scores had been correlated (0.90) with scores on Ware's Health Perception Questionnaire (Ware, 1976) "when patients with cancer were tested over time" (McCorkle, 1987, p. 254). Ragsdale and Morrow (1990) used the SDS as a measure of quality of life for persons with AIDS, AIDS-related complex, or positive serological tests for HIV. SDS scores were correlated (0.44 to 0.61) with scores on the Sickness Impact Profile (p. 357; see entry in this book).

PROCEDURE: The instrument takes 5 to 10 minutes to administer (McCorkle, 1987, p. 254). For each symptom item, respondents choose a statement and score that corresponds with how they have been feeling "lately." The five choices for each item on the scale have statements descriptive of degrees of distress, from *no distress* (1) to *extreme distress* (5).

SAMPLE ITEM: "Fatigue. (1) I am usually not tired at all; (2) I am occasionally rather tired; (3) There are frequently periods when I am quite tired; (4) I am usually very tired; (5) Most of the time, I feel exhausted" (McCorkle & Young, 1988).

SCORING: Total SDS scores, which may range from 13 to 65, are the sum of item scores.

SOURCE: The scale is available from Dr. McCorkle, who holds a copyright.

REFERENCES

McCorkle, R. (1987). The measurement of symptom distress. *Seminars in Oncology Nursing, 3,* 248-256.
McCorkle, R., Jepson, C., Malone, D., Lusk, E., Braitman, L., Buhler-Wilkerson, K., & Daly, J. (1994). The impact of posthospital home care on patients with cancer. *Research in Nursing and Health, 17,* 243-251.
McCorkle, R., & Young, K. (1978). Development of a symptom distress scale. *Cancer Nursing, 101,* 373-378.

McCorkle, R., & Young, K. (1988). *Symptom Distress Scale.* (Available from the authors at address listed above)

Ragsdale, D., & Morrow, J. R. (1990). Quality of life as a function of HIV classification. *Nursing Research, 39,* 355-359.

Ware, J. E., Jr. (1976). Scales for measuring general health perceptions. *Health Services Research, 11,* 396-415.

SYSTÈME DE MESURE DE L'AUTONOMIE FONCTIONNELLE (SMAF; FUNCTIONAL AUTONOMY MEASUREMENT SYSTEM)

AUTHORS: Réjean Hébert, R. Carrier, and A. Bilodreau
ADDRESS: Professor Réjean Hébert, MD, MPhil
            Centre de Recherche en Géronto-Gériatrie
            Sherbrooke Geriatric University Institute
            1036 rue Belvédère sud
            Sherbrooke, Québec J1H 4C4, Canada

DESCRIPTION: The SMAF is a 29-item instrument designed to evaluate the needs of individuals according to the World Health Organization's international classification of impairments, disabilities, and handicaps (World Health Organization, 1980). The authors synthesized prior instruments to obtain a global evaluative measure of the "disability-resources interval which corresponds to handicap" (Hébert, Carrier, & Bilodreau, 1988, pp. 293-294). The instrument may be used by nurses and social workers with community-dwelling elderly and in long-term care settings to obtain global scores for functional abilities in five areas: (a) activities of daily living, (b) mobility, (c) communication, (d) mental function, and (e) instrumental activities of daily living.

PSYCHOMETRIC PROPERTIES: The tool was validated in 1983 with a random sample of 146 home care and chronic care patients. Two hundred and ninety-two independent ratings were made by intermixed pairs of social workers and nurses. Twelve nurses and 18 social workers, selected at random, participated. Interrater reliability was demonstrated with weighted kappas ranging from 0.53 (Communication) to 0.76 (Instrumental Activities of Daily Living); mean weighted kappa was 0.75. Test-retest and interrater reliability for total SMAF scores was also verified with 90 subjects assessed within a

2-week interval. Intraclass correlations were 0.95 and 0.96, respectively (Desrosiers, Bravo, Hébert, & Dubuc, 1995). Scores on the SMAF were compared with a "validated measure of nursing care time" and were further validated by distinguishing between known groups with varying disabilities. The authors stated that the SMAF can be used to provide continuity in evaluating a patient who is slowly losing autonomy.

PROCEDURE: Administration of the SMAF is reported to take less than an hour; average time in trials was 42 minutes. Raters for trials were "given a brief explanation of the scale without specific training" (Hébert et al., 1988, p. 296). Reliabilities for initial ratings were compared with those obtained later and found not to have been "influenced by training." The authors concluded that administration "does not require any specific training" (p. 300). In addition to the rating for each item, the evaluator also rates whether the subject currently has the resources necessary to "overcome this disability," indicating where resources are the subject him- or herself, family members, neighbors, employees, aides, nurses, volunteers, or others. The predicted stability of the resource is also rated (i.e., whether the resource will lessen, increase, remain stable, or does not apply).

SAMPLE ITEM: Section 8: Mobility, Item 6: Negotiating Stairs

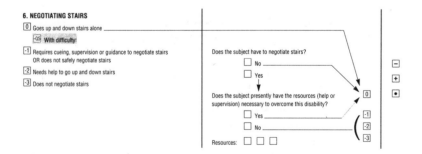

SCORING: For each item, rating is on a 4-point scale ranging from 0 (*complete autonomy or independent*), to –1 (*requires surveillance, stimula-*

tion or needs supervision), to –2 (*requires help*), to –3 (*totally dependent*). There is also a –0.5 rating for autonomy "with difficulty." The score indicating the greatest level of disability is –87. Eight items referring to IADLs and Item B-3 ("Walking outside") may be omitted when rating long-term care setting residents. The remaining 20 items will have a range from 0 to –3 for a total disability score of –60.

A care chart has also been constructed by the author so that assessments using the SMAF may be depicted visually.

SOURCE: The instrument, which is available from the authors, was developed in French. Versions in English, Dutch, and Spanish are also available.

REFERENCES

Desrosiers, J., Bravo, G., Hébert, R., & Dubuc, N. (1995). Reliability of the Revised Functional Autonomy Measurement System (SMAF) for epidemiological research. *Age and Ageing, 24,* 402-406.
Hébert, R., Carrier, R., & Bilodreau, A. (1988). The Functional Autonomy Measurement System (SMAF): Description and validation of an instrument for the measurement of handicaps. *Age and Ageing, 17,* 293-302.
World Health Organization. (1980). *International classification of impairments, disabilities and handicaps: A manual of classification relating to the consequences of disease.* Geneva: World Health Organization.

TAYLOR MANIFEST ANXIETY SCALE (TMAS)

AUTHOR: Janet Taylor Spence
ADDRESS: Janet Taylor Spence
            Alma Cowden Madden Professor
            Department of Psychology
            University of Texas at Austin
            Mezes Hall 330
            Austin, TX 78712

DESCRIPTION: The Taylor Manifest Anxiety Scale (TMAS) was originally developed "as a device for selecting subjects for experiments in human motivation" (Taylor, 1953, p. 290). The TMAS is a 50-item self-report instrument designed to evaluate the feelings, affects, and bodily symptoms characteristic of anxiety. The scale has been used in recent years in a variety of studies related to health care.

PSYCHOMETRIC PROPERTIES: From a pool of 200 Minnesota Multiphasic Personality Inventory (MMPI; Hathaway & McKinley, 1951) items, five clinician judges were asked by the author to designate "items indicative of manifest anxiety" (Taylor, 1953, p. 285). Sixty-five items about which these judges had high agreement were selected for testing. The items selected along with 135 additional buffer items judged "non-indicative of anxiety" were administered to samples of college students. The scale was further modified until 50 items that had high correlations with total anxiety scores were chosen for the final version. Correlations for students' test with retest scores were 0.89 for a 3-week retest interval, 0.82 for a 5-month interval, and 0.81 for 9- to 17-month intervals (pp. 285-286). With tests and retests, the author found that "both the relative position of the individual in the group and his absolute score tended to remain constant over relatively long periods of time" (p. 287). Distributions for scores of "neurotic and psychotic" persons ($n = 103$) and students ($n = 1,971$) were very different, however. Patients had significantly higher median scores (34 vs. 14.56) than students (p. 290). Fuller, Horii, and Connor (1992) reported internal consistency for the TMAS (alpha = 0.85) in a study of 88 graduate students. A shorter version of the TMAS was proposed by Bendig (1956).

PROCEDURE: The respondent completes a paper-and-pencil test prepared by the administrator in either a true-false or a Likert format.

SAMPLE ITEMS: "I am troubled by attacks of nausea," "I worry quite a bit over possible misfortunes," "I have had periods in which I lost sleep over worry," and "I am entirely self-confident" (Taylor, 1953, p. 286).

SCORING: There are two methods for scoring the TMAS. For the true-false version, 38 items are keyed true and 12 false; answers positive for anxiety are scored 1, and those in the nonanxious direction are scored 0. The total TMAS score is the sum of scores. When the other method, a 5-point scale, is used, endpoints for items are defined as *not at all true of me* and *very true of me*, with possible scores ranging from 1 to 5.

SOURCE: A copy of the instrument is available from the author. The TMAS items are also reprinted in Taylor (1953, Table 1). Items for a 24-item version of the scale, which the author considers "more focused," are indicated with asterisks in the copy of the TMAS she forwards.

REFERENCES

Bendig, A. W. (1956). The development of a short form of the Manifest Anxiety Scale. *Journal of Consulting Psychology, 20,* 384.

Fuller, B. F., Horii, Y., & Conner, D. A. (1992). Validity and reliability of nonverbal voice measures as indicators of stressor-provoked anxiety. *Research in Nursing and Health, 15,* 379-389.

Hathaway, S. R., & McKinley, J. C. (1951). *The Minnesota Multiphasic Personality Inventory manual.* New York: Psychological Corporation.

Taylor, J. A. (1953). A personality scale of manifest anxiety. *Journal of Abnormal and Social Psychology, 48,* 285-290.

TEST FOR SEVERE IMPAIRMENT (TSI)

AUTHORS: Marilyn Albert and Carolyn Cohen
ADDRESS: Marilyn Albert, PhD
            Department of Psychiatry
            Massachusetts General Hospital
            Boston, MA 02114

DESCRIPTION: The Test for Severe Impairment (TSI) was designed to quantify the abilities of individuals with severe cognitive impairment (Albert & Cohen, 1992). To be appropriate for these persons, the tasks for the test were designed to be nonthreatening, appealing, and easy to administer. To respond correctly, subjects are required to point, gesture, manipulate small objects, and use only a few verbal responses. The six subsections of the test assess "well learned motor performance, language comprehension, language production, immediate and delayed memory, general knowledge, and conceptualization" (p. 450).

PSYCHOMETRIC PROPERTIES: The authors administered the TSI to 40 nursing home residents who had achieved scores between 0 and 10 on the Mini-Mental State Examination (MMSE; see entry in this book). The test was administered to 19 of the 40 residents on two occasions at a 2-week interval. Scores for the total test at Time 1 were highly correlated (0.96) with those for

Time 2, and correlations of Time 1 and Time 2 subsection scores ranged from 0.74 to 0.97 (p. 450). The alpha coefficient for the overall TSI was 0.91 (p. 451). Mean score on the TSI was 14.6 ± 5.5, with a range from 3 to 23. The correlation between TSI scores and MMSE scores was 0.83. Residents with mid- to upper-range scores on the TSI had MMSE scores in the severely impaired range.

PROCEDURE: TSI administration takes approximately 10 minutes. Props needed for administration are small, readily available objects: colored pens, paper clips, a key, a comb, and a spool of thread.

SAMPLE ITEM: Motor Performance: A. Comb. Tester says, "Show me how you would use this comb" and hands subject a comb. If the subject correctly demonstrates combing, he or she scores 1 point (Albert & Cohen, 1992, p. 452).

SCORING: The maximum score for each subsection is 4. The maximum total score is 24.

SOURCE: The test format, which includes instructions for administration, is appended to Albert and Cohen (1992).

REFERENCE

Albert, M., & Cohen, C. (1992). The Test for Severe Impairment: An instrument for the assessment of patients with severe cognitive dysfunction. *Journal of the American Geriatrics Society, 40,* 449-453.

TIMED "UP AND GO" TEST (TUGT)

AUTHORS: Diane Podsiadlo and Sandra Richardson
ADDRESS: Diane Podsiadlo, BScPT
            Geriatric Day Hospital, S8 West
            Royal Victoria Hospital
            687 Pine Avenue West
            Montreal, Quebec H3A 1A1, Canada

DESCRIPTION: The Timed "Up and Go" is a simple performance measure of basic mobility skills, a modified timed version of the "Get Up and Go" test (Mathias, Nayak, & Isaacs, 1986). The timed version, which employs the maneuvers of everyday life, is quick, is easy to administer, and can be used by clinicians to screen and assess frail elderly persons. The authors suggested that "it is also an objective means of following functional change over time" (Podsiadlo & Richardson, 1991, p. 145).

PSYCHOMETRIC PROPERTIES: Podsiadlo and Richardson (1991) measured the validity of the test by hypothesizing relationships with other measures of balance (Berg Balance Scale; see entry in this book), gait speed (time taken to walk the middle 15 feet of a 20-meter course in meters/second), and functional capacity (Barthel Index; see entry in this book). They studied 60 geriatric patients in a day hospital (37 women and 23 men ranging in age from 60 to 90, with a mean age of 79.5) and 10 active healthy volunteers over 70 years of age. Correlations with balance (–0.81), gait speed (–0.61), and Barthel Index (–0.78) supported validity. The authors used intraclass correlation coefficients to show interrater (0.99) and test-retest (0.99) reliability. They cited case studies to demonstrate that the test was sensitive to both improving and declining function over time.

PROCEDURE: A line is drawn or a piece of tape is placed on the floor 3 meters from a chair. At the beginning of the test, the subject is seated with his or her back against a standard armchair (seat height approximately 46 cm) and with the customary walking aid (cane or walker, if any) available. The subject is instructed, "On the word 'go,' get up and walk at a comfortable and safe pace to that line (tape) on the floor; turn, return to the chair and sit down again." The subject has the opportunity to walk through the test once before being timed. The tester should not assist but should guard as needed.

SCORING: The score is the time in seconds taken to complete the test. Podsiadlo and Richardson (1991) used a watch with a second hand to time their subjects. The 10 healthy volunteers performed the test in 10 or fewer seconds. Scores lower than 20 seconds were associated with independence and ability to go outside alone, and scores above 30 seconds with dependency and inability to go out independently. In the 25% of the sample who scored between 20 and 29, functional ability was less definitive, with wide variations in balance and gait speed.

SOURCE: The procedure for the test is described in Podsiadlo and Richardson (1991).

REFERENCES

Mathias, S., Nayak, U. S. L., & Isaacs, B. (1986). Balance in elderly patients: The "get-up and go" test. *Archives of Physical Medicine and Rehabilitation, 67,* 387-389.

Podsiadlo, D., & Richardson, S. (1991). The timed "up & go": A test of basic functional mobility for frail elderly persons. *Journal of the American Geriatrics Society, 39,* 142-148.

TRIMS BEHAVIORAL PROBLEM CHECKLIST (TRIMS)

AUTHOR: George Niederehe

ADDRESS: George Niederehe, PhD
Head, Geriatric Treatment Research
National Institute of Mental Health
Parklawn Building, Room 18-105
5600 Fishers Lane
Rockville, MD 20857

DESCRIPTION: The TRIMS Behavioral Problem Checklist (TRIMS) is a "global measure of the severity of behavioral problems in dementia" (Niederehe, 1988, p. 772). It is a 52-item instrument that brings together items from several other existing instruments. The TRIMS was designed to be completed by caregivers who assess a range of behavioral problems exhibited by dementia patients in the areas of mental health and social roles. The profile emerging from responses to the items includes "symptoms, deficits, and interpersonal behaviors" as well as the caregiver's "emotional reaction to the behavior problems" (p. 771). There are six subscales: Cognitive Symptoms, Self-Care Deficits, Instrumental Activities of Daily Living, Dysphoric Mood, Acting-Out Behavior, and Inactivity/Withdrawal. The TRIMS may be administered in either of two formats, one referring to the respondent's "spouse" and the other to "your older relative."

PSYCHOMETRIC PROPERTIES: In initial testing, TRIMS responses from a sample of caregivers of dementia patients ($n = 42$) were compared with those of a control group of 25 relatives of cognitively "normal" elders. Internal consistency was demonstrated with alpha coefficients of 0.93 for the total scale and a range of 0.65 to 0.89 for subscales. For the dementia sample, the means for all subscales increased on retesting at approximately 1 year. Concurrent validity was supported by significant correlations between TRIMS subscale scores and scores on scales measuring similar behaviors (Niederehe, 1988, p. 772).

PROCEDURE: The TRIMS is a paper-and-pencil instrument. Respondents are instructed to reply about each behavior as to its frequency, duration, and the extent to which it upsets them. A separately paged key is provided for the respondent's easy reference. If the behavior does not occur, the response about frequency is 0, and the caregiver goes on to the next item. The duration scales may be omitted if a respondent is being retested.

SAMPLE ITEMS: "Having difficulty remembering how to do simple tasks," "Getting the present mixed up with past situations," "Wandering or getting lost," and "Being unable to handle money" (Niederehe, 1988, pp. 775-777).

SCORING: The frequency scale ranges between 0 (*problem does not occur*) and 4 (*problem occurs daily*). Both total TRIMS scores and subscale scores are calculated by summing scores for the relevant items and dividing by the number of those items. The caregiver's distress may be scored with a simple sum or by mean distress per behavior—that is, the sum divided by the number of behaviors. The latter score is seen as more likely to be independent of the volume of disturbing behaviors.

SOURCE: The instrument and instructions for administration and scoring appear in Niederehe (1988).

REFERENCE

Niederehe, G. (1988). TRIMS Behavioral Problem Checklist (BPC). *Psychopharmacology Bulletin, 24,* 771-778.

VIRO (VIGOR, INTACTNESS, RELATIONSHIP, ORIENTATION)

AUTHORS: Robert Kastenbaum and Sylvia Sherwood
ADDRESS: Robert Kastenbaum, PhD
            Arizona State University
            Adult Development/Aging Program
            Tempe, AZ 85287

DESCRIPTION: The VIRO is a technique for "assessing the interview behavior of elderly people" (Kastenbaum & Sherwood, 1972, p. 166). It has four dimensions, vigor, intactness, relationship, and orientation, and a total of 21 items. The technique may be used in a variety of interview situations, "including many that are conducted for purposes other than research" (p. 174). The VIRO was developed with the premise that "the interview itself constitutes a type of relevant data" (p. 166). The scale is not intended to differentiate among elders who are functioning well. Rather, it is useful for work with "more or less troubled or impaired elders" (p. 187). The technique may be used for repeated observations "without 'wearing out' or exercising a differential influence upon [the subject] at various points in time" (p. 173).

PSYCHOMETRIC PROPERTIES: The internal consistency of the VIRO was tested with two community samples ($n = 382$; $n = 140$) in Massachusetts (Kane & Kane, 1981). Alpha coefficients improved from 0.75 and 0.67 respectively to 0.81 and 0.72 when two items (repeating examiner's name and length of interview) were dropped from the scale (p. 94). The authors of the VIRO reported that it was "not difficult to train interviewers to rate reliably on the VIRO dimensions" and that the technique had "the potential to yield fairly reliable results" (Kastenbaum & Sherwood, 1972, p. 194). Perfect agreement, they said, was especially easy to obtain at the extremes of the scale. To improve reliability, they suggested that raters be trained in clinical interactions, simultaneously observing and independently rating an interview conducted by an experienced rater. Gender and group differences were found with longitudinal VIRO data. Newly admitted female patients tended to be rated lower in vigor than males, for example, and even with declining vigor and orientation, members of some ethnic groups maintained intactness longer than did others (Kastenbaum & Sherwood, 1972, p. 169).

PROCEDURE: Clinicians and investigators who use the VIRO must limit their ratings to actual observations, which requires that a clear distinction be made between the behavior itself and the explanation for the behavior. The first three observations are made during the first minute of contact. Bipolar variables are rated: vigorous/feeble, receptive/closed, and comfortable/in distress. The next six items are rated for the course of the whole interview: quite trustful/quite suspicious, high energy level/low energy level, fluent speech/minimal speech, keen attention/poor attention, controlled thought/ tangential-fragmented, and eager participation/reluctant participation. Three items are scored for their highest or peak score: keen self-perspective/no self-perspective, engrossment in own ideas and feeling/no engrossment, and engrossment in relationship/no engrossment in relationship. Another item is scored for the subject's behavior at the end of the session: Is he or she eager to continue, or to end the session? The orientation section of the VIRO, which is similar to other mental status exams and is sometimes used separately by investigators, may be used as part of the VIRO or omitted "altogether, as when it is feared that a period of direct questioning might interfere with other purposes of the interview" (Kastenbaum & Sherwood, 1972, p. 181). The initial three presentation variables are evaluated again when the session has ended.

SAMPLE ITEMS:

A. (3) Vigorous (0) Feeble. Vitality scale—hearty handshake, impression of capacity for effective, decisive movement vs. flaccid tonus, impression of weak, slow, ineffective movement. (Kastenbaum & Sherwood, 1972, p. 178)

H. (3) Engrossed in Own Ideas/Feelings (0) No Self-Engrossment. Animated, "alive" when talking about his life or opinions, as shown in sparkling or intense eyes, appropriate gestures, body posture, speech patterning—may also be shown by deeply reflective, inward-turning behavior, "lost in own thoughts and feelings" to such an extent that [evaluator's] presence seems momentarily ignored. These are two different patterns of self-engrossment vs. flat, neutral, transient, "uncommitted" behavioral and expressive "commentary" when talking about his life or opinions, not "caught up" in his internal life. Talks about himself in same, rather uninvolved way he talks about most everything else. (p. 180)

SCORING: Most items are scored on a 4-point scale, with higher scores indicating the more socially valued behavior. Total scores are computed using guidelines provided by the authors. A visual profile of scores for the four dimensions can be constructed by translating the scores into the same numerical scale (Kastenbaum & Sherwood, 1972, p. 188).

SOURCE: The VIRO scale, the Guide to Rating, and instructions to construct graphs for profile analysis appear in Kastenbaum & Sherwood (1972).

REFERENCES

Kane, R. A., & Kane, R. L. (1981). *Assessing the elderly.* Lexington, MA: D. C. Heath.
Kastenbaum, R., & Sherwood, S. (1972). VIRO: A scale for assessing the interview behavior of elderly people. In D. Kent, R. Kastenbaum, & S. Sherwood (Eds.), *Research planning and action for the elderly: The power and potential of social science* (pp. 166-200). New York: Behavioral Publications.

Glossary

Activities of daily living (ADLs) The basic ADLs are the self-maintenance functions of bathing, dressing, grooming, eating, transfer to and from a bed or chair, using the toilet, and continence. See **Instrumental Activities of Daily Living (IADLs).**

Alpha coefficient This coefficient of reliability, often reported as *Cronbach's alpha,* is a measure of the internal consistency of an instrument.

Biserial correlations or **point biserial correlations** Statistics that are used to estimate the associations between continuous and dichotomous variables.

Body mass index The index is the body weight adjusted for height. It is computed by dividing weight in kilograms by the square of height in meters.

Cathexis The process whereby mental or emotional energy is invested in another person, an idea, or an object.

Cluster analysis Procedures for multivariate analysis designed to investigate whether entities correspond enough to be grouped or clustered.

Coefficient of concordance A statistic that measures the extent of agreement for observations that have been ranked. When there is perfect agreement, the coefficient is 1; for perfect disagreement, it is 0.

Coefficient of reproducibility A coefficient that signifies the extent to which an investigator can reproduce the specific items with which a respondent agreed by knowing his or her score.

Comorbidity A disease process that coexists with another.

Concurrent validity The extent to which scores for one measure are correlated with scores on another measure known to be valid and observed at the same time.

Confirmatory factor analysis A statistical procedure used to test theories about the factors one expects to find.

221

Construct validity   The extent to which an instrument has operationalized a construct. It is usually estimated with simultaneous measurements of the similar or dissimilar variables that one would theoretically expect to be related or unrelated.

Content validity   The extent to which the items of an instrument are judged to represent the universe of content for the entity being measured.

Correlation   Two variables are said to be correlated when there is a tendency for one of them to vary as does the other. Correlation coefficients range from −1.00 (perfect negative correlation) to +1.00 (perfect positive correlation). The most widely used correlation is the *Pearson product moment* or *Pearson* r.

Criterion measure   A measure of the effect in a study, usually termed the *dependent variable.*

Discriminant analysis   A procedure used to classify cases categorically, using two or more predictor or independent variables.

Double-blind study   Procedure in an experiment where neither subjects nor those who administer the treatment condition are aware of a subject's assignment to either the experimental or the control group.

Empirically   Data gathered empirically are those based on observation or experience.

Face validity   The extent to which an instrument includes items that look (on the face of it) as if they will measure what they are intended to measure.

Factor analysis   A set of statistical procedures designed to reduce a large set of variables to smaller sets with the same properties. A factor is a cluster of highly correlated variables.

Guttman scale   These scales, also called *cumulative scales,* have a hierarchy of items of increasing intensity that relate to one concept.

Instrumental activities of daily living (IADLs)   Among these self-care abilities are meal preparation, transportation, shopping, managing money, doing housework (including laundry), and using the telephone.

Internal consistency   A measure of reliability of an instrument based on correlations between items or sections of a scale with other items or sections. The measure reflects the extent to which all parts of a scale are measuring the same entity.

Interrater reliability   The extent to which two or more independent observers agree in their ratings of some entity.

Intersubscale correlations   These correlations are performed to determine the extent to which subscales are measuring the same or different entities.

Interval scale   A scale with an interval level of measurement has units of measurement that can be rank ordered and are equally distant from each other. Such a scale does not indicate an absolute magnitude because it lacks a true zero.

Intraclass correlation coefficient (ICC) This coefficient signifies the extent to which two or more independent observers agree in their ratings of some entity.

Item-to-total-scale correlations These correlations are frequently computed when an instrument is being developed to determine the extent to which items are consistent with other items. These correlations are part of the calculations performed to measure the internal consistency of a scale.

Kappa statistics These statistics are coefficients of interjudge agreement for nominal scales representing the proportion of joint judgments where there is agreement after agreement by chance has been removed.

Known groups Samples with known attributes whose scores on a measure may therefore be used to estimate validity of an instrument.

Kuder-Richardson Formulas 20 and 21 (KR-20) Procedures to estimate reliability, used for tests with nominal levels of measurement and forced-choice responses.

Likert scale These scales have an array of declarative statements about which the respondent is asked for the extent of agreement or disagreement.

Longitudinal studies Studies in which investigators collect data on two or more occasions over time.

Mann-Whitney *U* test A statistical test of difference between groups, used when observations have been rank ordered, or measured with ordinal scales.

Median The point in a distribution of scores below which fall 50% of the scores.

Multitrait-multimethod techniques Statistical procedures used to estimate construct validity by analyzing variables with multiple measures.

Nursing diagnosis According to the North American Nursing Diagnosis Association, a clinical judgment about individual, family, or community responses to actual or potential health problems/life processes. Nursing diagnoses provide the basis for selection of nursing interventions to achieve outcomes for which the nurse is accountable.

Ordinal rating An observation of a variable that puts it in a rank order.

Orthogonal Uncorrelated.

Praxis The ability to plan and execute coordinated movements.

Predictive validity The extent to which observations made at a given time are capable of predicting subsequent occurrences.

Prospective study A clinical or epidemiological study of factors encountered through time to investigate the presumed effects of presumed causes.

Q-sort   A method by which observers order or sort cards into a number of piles representing selected points on a bipolar continuum.

Ratio scale   A level of measurement that includes equal intervals and a true zero.

Reliability coefficients   Statistics signifying the extent to which an instrument measures accurately and precisely. Reliable measurement is dependable and consistent over time.

Response bias   A systematic pattern of responding to items, such as always agreeing or always disagreeing despite the item content.

Retrospective study   Analysis of data gathered in the past to describe or explain a current phenomenon.

Reverse scoring   Scoring in reverse is necessary when investigators construct items to counteract response bias.

Scoring algorithms   A set of scoring rules.

Sensitivity   One meaning of this term refers to the extent to which an instrument can detect change. *Sensitivity* also refers to the extent to which the presence of a condition is correctly identified by an instrument. It is reported as the proportion of individuals who have a condition and also have a positive test for that condition. See **Specificity.**

Significance or significant differences   Investigators accept statistical levels of significance at probability levels such as 0.05, 0.01, and 0.001. If results are supported at $p < 0.01$, it means that there is less than 1 chance in 100 that the results could have occurred by chance.

Social desirability   This is a biased response pattern used by persons who give answers they believe will be socially acceptable.

Spearman-Brown formula   The formula can be used to calculate the extent to which reliability could be improved when the number of observations is increased.

Spearman rank correlations   This correlation is also called *Spearman's rho*. It is a statistic that shows the extent of relationship between ordinal variables.

Specificity   The extent to which the absence of a condition is correctly identified by an instrument. It is reported as the proportion of individuals who do not have a condition and who also have a negative test for that condition. See **Sensitivity.**

Split-half analysis   A method for checking the internal consistency of an instrument. Scores from one half of the instrument are correlated with scores for the other half. Investigators split responses from either odd and even items or the first and last halves of a test.

Tardive dyskinesia   An involuntary movement disorder.

Test-retest reliability   An estimate of the extent to which an instrument can elicit the same results in repeated administrations to a stable population.

Variance   The measure of the dispersion or spread of scores in a distribution.

Visual analogue scale   A vertical or horizontal line, often 100 mm in length, and anchored with terms describing polar extremes of a phenomenon, such as anxiety, confusion, dyspnea, mood, or pain. Subjects rate the intensity of their experience of the phenomenon on the line.

z **score**   A commonly used standard score where the mean is 0, and the standard deviation is 1. A *z* score of 2 represents a score that is 2 standard deviations above the mean.

Index of Abbreviations and Acronyms

ABRS	Agitated Behavior Rating Scale
ABS	Affect Balance Scale; see *MUNSH*
AD	Alzheimer's disease
ADAS	Alzheimer's Disease Assessment Scale
ADL	Activities of Daily Living
AGECAT	A computerized psychiatric diagnostic system and case nomenclature for elderly subjects developed in Britain.
AIMS	Abnormal Involuntary Movement Scale; the acronym is also used for the Arthritis Impact Measurement Scales
AIMS2	Arthritis Impact Measurement Scales, Revised
ASI	Anxiety Status Inventory
BANS-S	Bedford Alzheimer Nursing Severity Scale
BARS	Brief Agitation Rating Scale
BAS-DEP	Depression Scale of the Brief Assessment Scale
BBS	Berg Balance Scale
BC-SC	Body Cathexis Scale
BCRS	Brief Cognitive Rating Scale
BDI	Beck Depression Inventory
BHS	Beck Hopelessness Scale
BI	Barthel Index
BOHSE	Kayser-Jones Brief Oral Health Status Examination
BRADEN	Braden Scale
BRS	Behavior Rating Scale of the CAPE
BURDEN	Burden Interview
BWBD	Body Worries and Body Discomforts Tests
CADET	See *FROMAJE*
CAGE	CAGE Questionnaire
CAM	Confusion Assessment Method
CAPE	Clifton Assessment Procedures for the Elderly
CARE	Comprehensive Assessment and Referral Evaluation; see *PADL*
CAS	Cognitive Assessment Scale

CASI	Cognitive Abilities Screening Instrument
CCSE	Cognitive Capacity Screening Examination
CDR	Washington University Clinical Dementia Rating Scale
CHQ	Chronic Heart Failure Index Questionnaire; see *CRQ*
CINAHL	Cumulative Index to Nursing and Allied Health Literature
CL	Cantril's Ladder or Ladder Scale
CLOCK	Clock Test
CLOCS	Comprehensive Level of Consciousness Scale
CMAI	Cohen-Mansfield Agitation Inventory
CPS	Minimum Data Set (MDS) Cognitive Performance Scale
CRA	Caregiver Reaction Assessment
CRBRS and CR	Crichton Royal Behavioural Rating Scale and Confusion Rating
CRQ	Chronic Respiratory Disease Questionnaire
CSDD	Cornell Scale for Depression in Dementia
DAFS	Direct Assessment of Functional Status
DAS	Death Anxiety Scale
DAT-DS	Discomfort Scale
DBRI	Dysfunctional Behavior Rating Instrument
DDS	Death Depression Scale; see *DAS*
DIS-Co	Dyskinesia Identification System—Coldwater; see *DISCUS*
DISCUS	Dyskinesia Identification System: Condensed User Scale
DMAS	Dementia Mood Assessment Scale
DMAS17	Mood subscale of the DMAS
DMAS18-24	Dementia Severity subscale of the DMAS
DS	Blessed Dementia Scale
DSI	Depression Status Inventory
DSS	Depressive Signs Scale
DUHP	Duke-UNC Health Profile
DUKE	Duke Health Profile
EBAS-DEP	Even Briefer Assessment Scale for Depression
EIIC	Everyday Indicators of Impaired Cognition
ERIC	Educational Resources Information Center of the U.S. Department of Education
ESDS	Enforced Social Dependency Scale
ESS	Epworth Sleepiness Scale
ETS	Educational Testing Service
EWBS	Existential Well-Being Scale; see *SWBS*
FACES	Faces Scale
FAQ	Functional Activities Questionnaire
FAST	Functional Assessment Staging System
FES	Falls Efficacy Scale
FPQLI	Ferrans and Powers Quality of Life Index
FR	Functional Reach

MSLT	Multiple Sleep Latency Test; see *ESS*
MUNSH	Memorial University of Newfoundland Scale of Happiness
n	Number in a subsample
N	Number in a total sample
NAs	Nursing assistants, nurse's aides, nursing attendants
NCHS	National Center for Health Statistics
NEECHAM	Neecham Confusion Scale
NHANES	National Health and Nutrition Examination Survey
NHBPS	Nursing Home Behavior Problem Scale
NIMH	National Institute of Mental Health
NOSGER	Nurses' Observation Scale for Geriatric Patients
NRI	Nutritional Risk Index
OCLC	Online Computer Library Center
PAB	Physically Aggressive Behavior subscale; see *RAS*
PADL	Performance activities of daily living
PAI	Preadmission Acuity Inquiry
PGCMS	Philadelphia Geriatric Center Morale Scale, Revised
PRI	Pain Rating Index; see *MPQ*
PSQ	Perceived Stress Questionnaire
PSQI	Pittsburgh Sleep Quality Index
PSS	Perceived Stress Scale
PULSES	PULSES Profile
RAGE	Rating Scale for Aggressive Behavior in the Elderly
RAI	Resident Assessment Instrument; see *CPS*
RAS	Ryden Aggression Scales, Form 1 and Form 2
RBS	Roberts Balance Scale
RDRS2	Rapid Disability Rating Scale-2
RNs	Registered nurses
RPE	Rating of Perceived Exertion; see *Borg Scale*
RS	Resilience Scale
RSE	Rosenberg Self-Esteem Scale
RWBS	Religious Well-Being Scale; see *SWBS*
SAB	Sexually Aggressive Behavior subscale; see *RAS*
SAS	Self-Rating Anxiety Scale
SCAG	Sandoz Clinical Assessment-Geriatric
SCDA	Situational Control of Daily Activities
SD	Standard deviation
SDQ	Social Disability Questionnaire
SDS	Symptom Distress Scale
SERENITY	Serenity Scale
SGSS	Stokes/Gordon Stress Scale
SIP	Sickness Impact Profile
SIP-NH	Sickness Impact Profile for Nursing Homes

Index of Instrument Authors

Index of Nursing Diagnoses

To assist readers, some nursing diagnoses are listed twice in this index. For example, both *Adjustment, impaired* and *Impaired adjustment* are listed.

Index of Subject Terms

Index of Instrument Titles

About the Authors

Sarah R. Beaton, PhD, RN, is Associate Professor of Nursing at Lehman College, The City University of New York, the Bronx, NY. She has taught nursing research, gerontological nursing and psychiatric-mental health nursing. From 1990 to 1994, she was consultant for nursing research and nursing education at Coler Memorial Hospital of the New York City Health and Hospitals Corporation. From 1993 to 1995, she was coinvestigator for a study, "Nursing Diagnoses and Related Outcomes in Long-Term Care," funded by the National Institute for Nursing Research (5RO1 NR02912-02). She has studied the life stories of older women and has integrated fiction about aging into gerontological nursing courses.

Susan A. Voge, MSLS, MBA, is Assistant Professor, Reference Librarian, and Coordinator of Library Instruction at Lehman College, The City University of New York, the Bronx, NY. She is consultant to a consumer health Internet Web site (www.noah.cuny.edu) sponsored by the City University of New York, the New York Public Library, and the New York Academy of Medicine. Teaching the use of the library and consumer health information are her main research interests. Her article "Searching Electronic Databases to Locate Tests and Measures" appeared in *Reference Services Review* in 1994.